Patient Guide to Hair Loss & Hair Restoration

D.J. Verret, MD

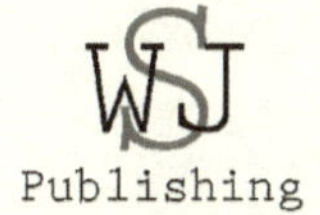

WJ Sonnier Publishing
Plano, TX

WJ Sonnier Publishing
6545 Preston Road, Suite 200
Plano, TX 75024
972.608.0100 voice, 972.473.7828 fax

Ordering Information:
To order additional copies, contact your local bookstore, visit www.WJSonnier.com, or call 972.608.0100.

ISBN: 978-0-578-01492-0

Library of Congress Control Number: 2009924300

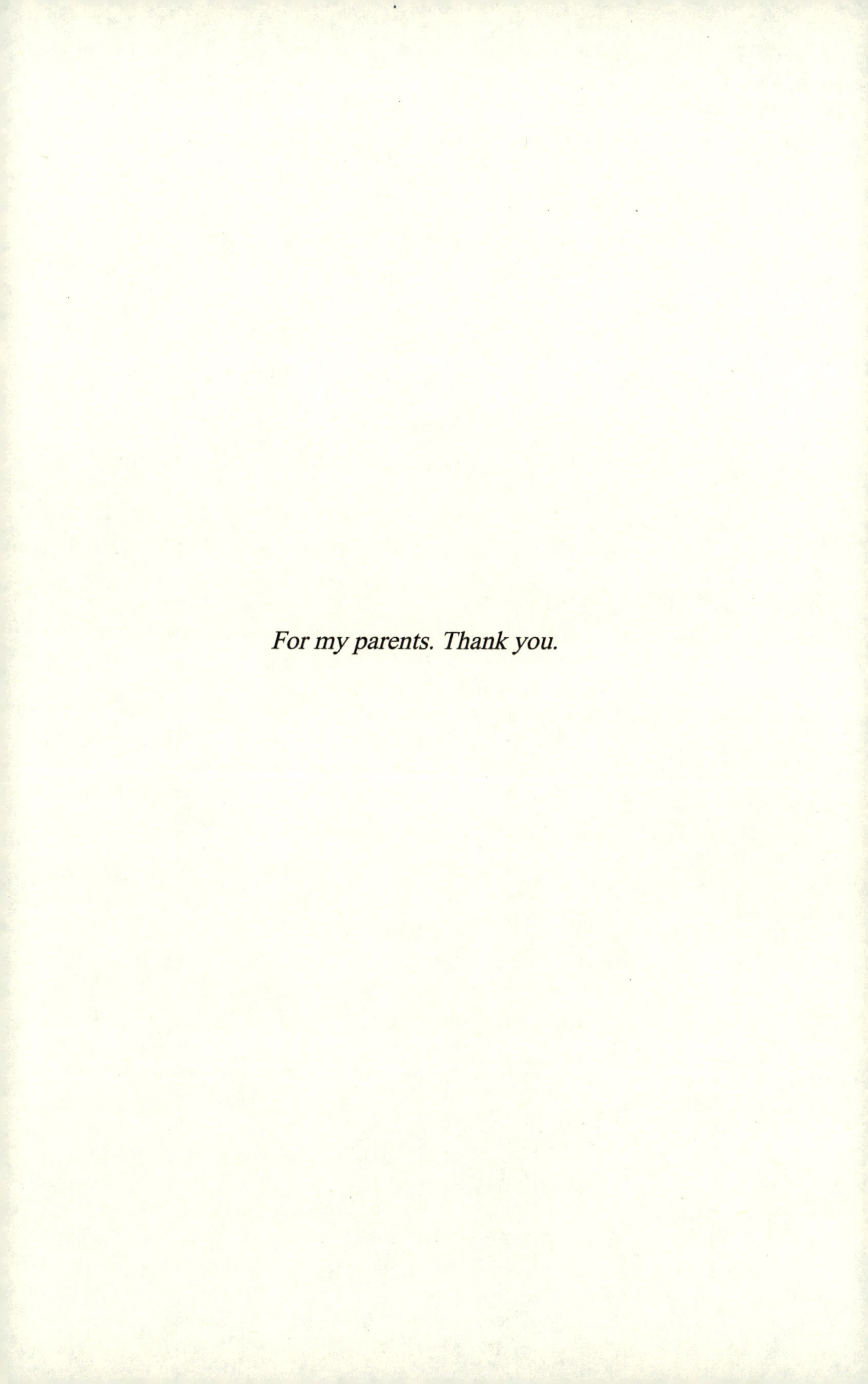

For my parents. Thank you.

Disclaimer

This book is designed to provide information about the subject matter covered. It is not the purpose of the book to reprint all the information that is available on the topics and the reader is urged to read all available material before undertaking any procedure.

Every effort has been made to make this book as complete and accurate as possible. Even with this effort, there may be errors in content and typographical errors. Therefore, this text should be used as a general guide and starting point for research. The information contained in the book is accurate as of the date of publication. Mention of a particular medication or device is not an endorsement of the item. Similarly, omission of a medication or device is not meant to indicate inferiority of the device or medication.

The purpose of this book is to educate. The author and WJ Sonnier Publishing shall have neither liability nor responsibility to any person or entity with respect to any loss or damage caused, directly or indirectly by the information contained in this book.

Contents

Part I

Introduction

Hair loss has been a problem for as long as humans have existed. For most of that time, humans have also tried treatments for hair loss. While the understanding of the hair loss process has progressed tremendously, human ability to stop the process or reverse its effects 100% have not progressed.

Hair loss, while not life threatening, can certainly be ego threatening. Numerous studies have illustrated the psychological impact of hair loss on adults as well as children. Societal stereotypes still exist which portray bald people as less virile and weaker than those with a full head of hair.

Hair loss affects 35 million men and 21 million women in the United States alone. It is estimated that 40% of men have some amount of noticeable hair loss by age 35 and 65% of men have some amount of noticeable hair loss by age 60. Hair loss treatment is big business. Many companies have rushed to fill the vacuum left by our inability to come up with a sure fire method for hair loss prevention and hair restoration. Unfortunately, not all of these promises of hair restoration are genuine.

As the second book in the Patient Guide series, the *Patient Guide to Hair Loss & Hair Restoration* continues the tradition of objective information for patients thinking about cosmetic procedures. This book includes information about the causes of hair loss as well as surgical and non-surgical methods for treating hair loss. As with any condition, it is not a substitute for the counsel of a knowledgeable physician.

I wish you well on your journey toward facial aesthetic improvement.

D.J. Verret, MD
Facial Plastic & Reconstructive Surgery

Part II

History of Hair Loss

Hair loss has been noted by people for centuries. The earliest mention of hair loss is in the Bible where many different passages have reference to hair, balding, or graying. Proverbs even mentions the virtues of gray hair in 16:31 "Grey hair is a crown of splendor; it is attained by a righteous life."

In 1500 BC Assyria, law dictated hairstyles according to social position and occupation. Baldness was covered by wigs and there were many treatments for hair loss. The Ebers Papyrus of ancient Egypt circa 1553 BC, the oldest medical text found, described a prescription for hair loss. The mixture was made of iron, red lead, onions, alabaster, and honey. Patients were instructed to swallow the potion after first reciting a magical invocation to the sun god.

Hippocrates, the Father of Medicine, in 400 BC was interested in hair loss. He was the first to note a connection between hair loss and the sexual organs. When studying eunuchs, Hippocrates noted that they did not experience hair loss. These results were echoed in 1995 in a study by Duke University researchers. As we understand now, it is because eunuchs do not produce dihydrotestosterone. Suffering from hair loss, he also created potions to try to grow hair. He actually prescribed a mixture of cumin, pigeon droppings, horseradish and beetroots, to help prevent hair loss. The term for one form of hair loss, alopecia areata, is actually derived from the Greek word for "mangy fox".

Roman society was believed to be the first to have professional barbers in 303 BC. Social standards mandated hair grooming and balding was thought to be an affliction which was actively treated. The 'comb over' tradition is originally credited to Julius Caesar. It is said that to cover his thinning hair, he wore a wreath on his head and grew his hair long in the back to comb it over his balding areas of the scalp. Cleopatra is said to have treated Caesar with a tonic of ground horse teeth, deer marrow, bear grease, and charred mice.

Current technologies for hair restoration surgeries pick up in the twentieth century. A Japanese dermatologist, Dr. Okuda, was the first to describe hair transplant techniques in 1939. Unfortunately he died during World War II and his work was lost. The next evolution of the technology came in 1959 in the United States with Dr. Norman Orentreich who described full size hair transplant grafting. Further refinement was undertaken to achieve today's gold standard of surgical restoration, follicular unit grafting.

As discussed in later chapters, many other cultures attempted treatment for hair loss. Unfortunately, to this day, none have proven successful at preventing hair loss 100% of the time. Though our understanding of hair loss has progressed tremendously, our ability to stem the loss has not.

Part III

Psychology of Hair Loss

Though hair loss is not a life threatening condition, studies have illustrated that hair loss can have a significant effect on quality of life. Patients can experience additional stress from concern over hair loss which in turn can add to future hair loss. Many studies have been performed which reinforce the fact that hair loss can take a psychological toll on the person with the loss and carry negative stereotypes.

According to the Hair Loss Learning Center web site, a 1971 study done with a picture of the same person with different degrees of baldness drawn in was shown to 60 people. Respondents indicated that the person with the balding head of hair was weak, dull, and inactive. The same person with a bald head of hair was rated as unkind, bad, and ugly. Yet the same person with a full head of hair was rated as handsome, virile, strong, active, and sharp.

In a 2006 Turkish study, both balding and non-balding males were questioned about the psychological and social implications of balding. A majority of the respondents indicated that hair loss would produce psychologically negative results. The respondents indicated a possible negative effect on other family members, relationships with the opposite sex, and occupation/academic life.

The most recent study to demonstrate a negative psychological impact from hair loss was published in Britain in 2009. The study consisted of 171 women and 43 men with hair loss who were given several standardized surveys concerning quality of life measures. The results showed a decrease in quality of life for several measures and the results were worse for women than for men.

Unfortunately adults are not the only patients affected by hair loss. Children also suffer from hair loss and the psychological impact should not be minimized. Several programs have been set up to help children deal with hair loss including ones which provide wigs for children for little to no cost.

Part IV

Anatomy & Physiology

Understanding hair loss begins with understanding hair growth. This includes understanding the anatomy of the hair as well as the hair growth cycle. What is termed a 'hair' is actually a complex unit of hair shaft, follicle, and additional skin appendages. A developing fetus has all of the hair follicles that will form by week 22 – one million on the head, 100,000 on the scalp, and a total of 5 million on the body. As a person grows, no additional follicles will grow and if a follicle dies or is damaged, it will not regrow.

The hair shaft is the part of the hair that is seen. It is composed of dead cells of fused keratin and is three layers. The outer layer of the hair shaft, the cuticle, consists of overlapping cells arranged like shingles. This layer connects to a portion of the follicle and helps to form a continuous layer. The middle layer, the hair cortex, is the majority of the hair shaft and grows outward with keratinization. The innermost layer, the medulla, is sometimes absent and is often difficult to see, even with microscopy.

The follicle is the part of the hair which exists below the skin which grows the shaft. Follicles are very complex structures which change during various portions of the hair cycle as well as various parts of the body. The follicle can be divided into three segments: lower, middle, and upper. The upper segment extends from the skin to the top of the sebaceous duct. The middle segment extends from the sebaceous duct to the insertion of the erector pili muscle. The lower segment contains the bulb and extends down from the insertion of the erector pili muscle.

The erector pili muscle is responsible for making hair stand on end when cold or scared. The bulb is the base of the hair follicle and contains the living part of the hair. Part of the bulb, the papilla, contains small blood vessels called capillaries which provide nutrients to the growing hair. The papilla extends like a finger into the base of the hair. The cells in the bulb are the most rapidly dividing in the body, every 2-3 days. The follicle is composed of two sheaths – an inner and outer. These provide the growing hair with support.

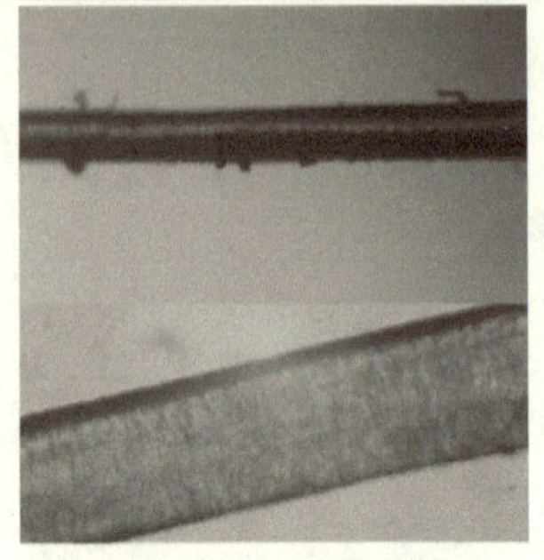

Magnified view of hair. Courtesy of microscopeworld.com

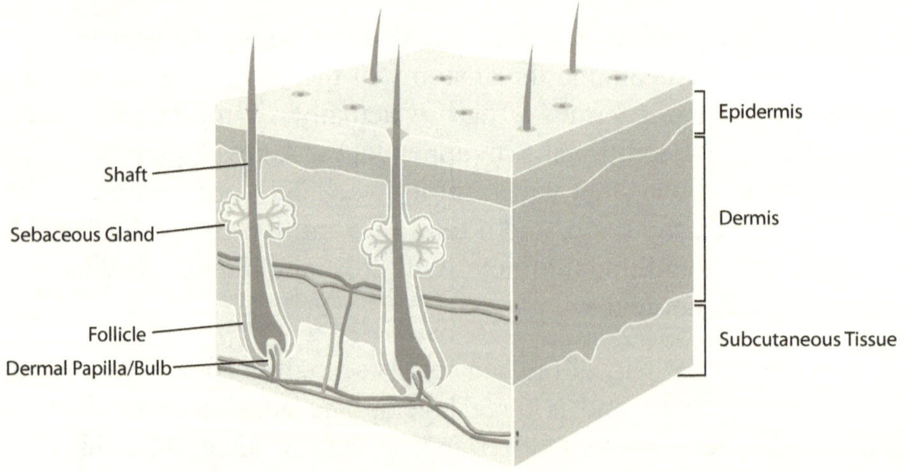

There are three types of follicles: vellus hair follicles located over most of the body; terminal hair follicles located on the scalp, groin, beard, axilla and several other areas; and sebaceous hair follicles located on the scalp, face, beard, chest, back, axilla, and groin. Growth of the follicles is influenced by factors in the dermis as well as androgens because of type II androgen receptors on the follicles. If damaged or killed, follicles will not regenerate like other skin layers.

Structures which surround the follicle are termed appendages. These include sebaceous glands which are attached to some of the follicles by a short duct. Sebaceous glands, or oil glands, are activated during puberty and secrete through the duct into follicles or sometimes directly onto the skin's surface. The secretion, called sebum, helps to lubricate and keep hair healthy. Some hairs also have an apocrine gland which provides scent.

Hair growth goes through a cycle with three identified stages - catagen (transitional phase), telogen (resting phase), and anagen (growing phase). Approximately eighty-five percent to ninety percent of hairs are in the anagen phase, two to three percent in catagen, and ten percent to fifteen percent are in the telogen phase at any point in time. In the scalp, the anagen phase lasts between 2 to 6 years, catagen between 2 to 3 weeks, and telogen between 2 to 3 months. In other areas of the body, anagen may be as short as 4 months long.

In the anagen phase, scalp hair grows approximately 0.35mm per day or about 6 inches per year but slows with age. Length of hair corresponds to the amount of time in the anagen phase. Scalp hair remains in the anagen phase longer than hair in other parts of the body. This explains why hair on the head is longer than hair on other parts of the body, such as the eyebrows which only spend 30-45 days in the anagen phase.

Catagen is the period of transition between the anagen phase and the telogen phase. Less than 1% of hairs are in this 2-3 week period at any one time. Changes take place in the structure of the hair follicle and at the end of catagen, telogen phase is entered.

Telogen phase is the resting phase of the hair follicle. At the end of the telogen phase, the hair follicles will reenter anagen phase and start growing again. Approximately 5-10% of scalp hair is in the telogen phase at any one time and these follicles are randomly distributed. It is during telogen that hair is normally shed. Approixmately 25-100 hairs are normally shed each day, more with shampooing.

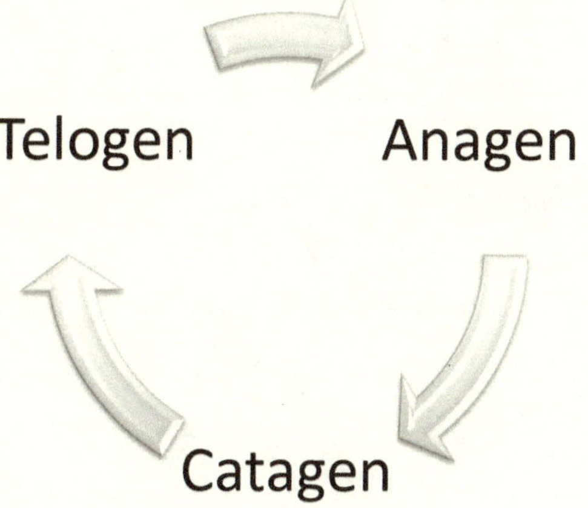

Additional Web References

http://dermatology.about.com/cs/hairanatomy/a/hairbiology.htm
http://emedicine.medscape.com/article/835470-overview

Both references have excellent introductions to hair anatomy and the hair cycle. The emedicine article is a bit more clinician oriented.

Part V

Causes of Hair Loss

There are many different causes of hair loss all with different treatments. Some of the causes are due to medical reasons and some are multifactorial. It is imperative that patients undergo evaluation by a trained physician before embarking on any kind of treatment regimen. Some causes of hair loss require medical treatment and delaying treatment can unnecessarily increase hair loss.

Androgenic Alopecia

The most common cause of hair loss, or alopecia, is often referred to as male patterned baldness. More appropriately, this condition is termed androgenic alopecia, and can effect women as well as men. The exact prevalence of androgenic alopecia is unknown. Several studies have reported a greater than 95% incidence in Caucasian men. The incidence increases with age and shows ethnic differences. Estimates have said that 25% of men aged 25 years have some degree of clinically apparent androgenic alopecia and over 40% of men will develop androgenic alopecia at some point in their life. Androgenic alopecia appears to effect Caucasians most often, followed by East Indians, Asians, and Africans.

The development of androgenic alopecia is dependent on several factors including endocrine and genetic factors but is ultimately due to the effect of androgens, such as testosterone and its byproducts, on hair follicles. In the body, testosterone is broken down into dihydrotestosterone by an enzyme called 5-alpha reductase. Testosterone is also broken down by another set of enzymes called the aromatase enzyme into estradiol and androstenedione. Therefore, an excess of 5-alpha reductase or a deficiency of aromatase can lead to excess dihydrotestosterone(DHT) production. Testosterone influences axillary and public hair growth, whereas DHT affects beard growth and scalp hair, areas which show androgenic alopecia.

In order to be effected by any hormone, a cell must have a receptor on the outside of the cell which is able to connect with that hormone. In the case of the scalp, hair on the top and crown of the head have receptors for DHT while hair on the back and sides of the scalp do not. This knowledge serves as the basis for current hair restoration transplant techniques. Because they do not have DHT receptors, hair on the back and sides of the head will not fall out in patients suffering from androgenic alopecia. When transplanted to a new site, the hair will not gain DHT receptors and will start to grow as if nothing had happened. The transplanted follicle will not be susceptible to DHT that the native hair was.

Androgenic alopecia results from progressive shortening of the anagen cycle with resultant decreased time for hair growth. The hair will transform from a thick pigmented hair to a fine, colorless, almost invisible hair. The length of time in telogen increases leading to a reduction in total hair density.

Hair loss usually begins with the frontoparietal scalp and then the vertex. Female-pattern baldness is similar but more diffuse, without complete baldness and maintaining the anterior hairline. Androgenic alopecia appears to be genetically determined and its development is related to age and presence of hormones and the corresponding receptors.

The exact genetic basis of androgenic alopecia has not been determined. Several theories and genes have been suggested but none have been definitely proven. It appears that several genes are responsible for androgenic alopecia. The risk of developing androgenic alopecia increases with a family history in a patient's father, mother, or maternal grandfather.

Diagnosis is fairly easy given an appropriate history and hair loss pattern and no further testing is generally done. For female patients with evidence of androgen hormone excess, such as inappropriate hair growth in other areas, further testing may be necessary.

Alopecia Areata

The second most common form of alopecia is alopecia areata. This form of hair loss results in rapid loss of hair in circular or oval patches. It can progress to encompass the whole scalp, which is termed alopecia totalis, or the entire body, alopecia universalis. It may be episodic or persistent. There is no definite reason why alopecia areata develops, but there is a genetic predisposition, and popular opinion favors an autoimmune disorder. Alopecia areata only affects 0.1% of people and equally effects men and women. Diagnosis is made by microscopic examination of a scalp biopsy in the effected area.

Alopecia areata will generally resolve within six months to a year. Should it persist for longer, the chance of recovery is minimal. The condition will recur in approximately one third of patients. Medical conditions including thyroid abnormalities, vitiligo, and pernicious anemia can accompany alopecia areata. In addition to diagnosing and treating any accompanying medical conditions, medications can be used to treat the hair loss. These medications include steroids and other immunomodulators. Topical, subcutaneous injections, or system medications may be used alone or in combination. One study even suggested hypnotherapy as a successful treatment for alopecia areata. Unfortunately some patients end up resorting to hairpieces or other methods of covering the hair loss because of severe cases not responsive to therapy.

Telogen Effluvium

Approximately 3 months after surgery, childbirth, crash dieting, and other stressful events, hair can enter an extended resting cycle referred to as telogen effluvium. Usually <50% of the scalp is affected and recovery is complete once the triggering event is resolved. Full recovery take takes six months or longer to occur.

Medications

A wide range of medications can cause hair loss. The most widely known are chemotherapy drugs but other more common drugs including blood thinners and Vitamin A can cause hair loss. After taking the medications, hair growth is abruptly interrupted and growing hairs are shed after 1-4 weeks. This form of hair loss rapidly affects 80-90% of the scalp but complete recovery can be expected once the medication is stopped. Listed below are some of the drugs which can cause hair

Medications Associated with Hair Loss

ACE inhibitors
- captopril
- enalapril
- moexipril
- ramipril

Allopurinol
Amiodarone
Amphetamines
Analgesics/antinflammatories
- ibuprofen
- indomethacin
- naproxen

Androgen
Anticoagulants
- coumadin
- dextran
- heparin and derivatives

Antiepileptics
- carbamazepine
- hydantoines
- troxidone
- valproic acid
- vigabatrin

Antipsychotics
- flupenthixol decanoate
- fluphenazine decanoate

Antithyroid drugs
- carbimazole
- iodine
- thiouracil

Appetite suppressants
Aromatase inhibitors
- fadrozole
- 4-OHA
- vorozole

Benzimidazoles
- albendazole
- mebendazole

Beta-blockers
- levobunolol
- metoprolol
- nadolol
- propanolol
- timolol

Bromocriptine
Buspiron
Butyrrophenones
Cantharidine
Cholestyramine
Chloramphenicol
Cidofovir
Cimetidine
Clonazepam
Clotrimazole
Colchicine
Oral Contraceptives
Danazol
Diclofenac
Dixyrazine
Dyazoxide
Ethambutol
Etionamide
Gentamicin
Glatiramer acetate
Glibenclamide
Gold salts
G-CSF
Haloperidol
Hypocholesterolemic drugs
- clofibrate
- fenofibrate

Immunoglobulins
Indandiones
Indinavir
Interferons
Isonicotinic acid hydrazide
Leflunomide
Levodopa
Lithium
Maprotilene
Mesalazine
Methyldopa
Methysergide
Methyrapone
Minoxidile
Nicotinic acid
Nitrofurantoin
Octreotide
Olanzapine
Pentosone polysulphate
Phenindione
Piroxicam
Potassium thiocyanate
Pyridostigmine
Radiation (<700 Gy)
Retinol (vitamin A)
Retinoids
- acitretin
- etretinate
- isotretinoin

Risperidone
Salicylates
Serotonin uptake inhibitors
- fluoxetin
- paroxetine

Spironolactone
Sulphasalazine
Tamoxifene
Terbinafine
Terfenadine
Thiamphenicol
Thrimetadione
Thyroxine
Tocopherol (vitamin E)
Trazodone
Triazoles
- fluconazole
- itraconazole

Tricyclic antidepressants
- amytriptiline
- desipramine
- doxepin
- imipramine
- maprotiline

Triparanol
Vasopressin

Medications Associated with Hair Change

Hair Graying	*Hair Darkening*	*Change in texture*
Althesin	Indinavir	Chemotherapy Agents
Benzoylperoxide	Chemotherapy agents	Indinavir
Butyrophenones	Arsenic	Interferon
Chloroquine	Bromocriptine	Lithium
Cyclosporine A	Carbidopa	Retinoids
Etretinate	Diazoxide	Valproic Acid
Hydroquinone	Estrogens	
Interferon-a	Minoxidil	
Mephenesine	Para-aminobenzoic acid	
Phenols	Prostaglandin analogs	
Phenylthiourea	Radiation therapy	
Triparanol	Tamoxifen	
	Verapamil	
	Zidovudine	

loss. It is not an exhaustive list but includes many of the most common offenders.

Trichotillomania

The most common cause of childhood alopecia is trichotillomania. It is an impulsive disorder in which the patient must pull their hair. Onset is in the early teens. Treatment relies on counseling, behavior modification techniques, and hypnosis. Once the behavior is stopped, the hair will generally regrow as long as scarring has not occurred.

Fungal Infections

Fungal infections of the scalp can cause hair loss in prepubertal patients. Diagnosis of fungal infection is made with a potassium hydroxide slide under a microscope or culture of the fungus which can take quite some time. Once the diagnosis is made, antifungal medications either by mouth and/or applied to the scalp are used to treat the infections.

Nutritional Deficiencies

Nutritional deficiencies can present as hair loss. Generalized malnutrition, zinc deficiency, and iron deficiency are the most common deficiencies causing hair loss. The loss is generalized over the entire body. Once the deficiency is corrected, the loss will generally resolve.

Underlying Disease

Hair loss may occur as part of an underlying disease. Many diseases are associated with hair loss including lupus, diabetes, syphilis, sarcoidosis, lichen planus follicularis, and thyroid disorders. A small patch of hair loss may indicate a skin cancer such as a basal cell carcinoma, squamous cell carcinoma, or other skin cancer. Since hair loss may be an early sign of a disease, it is important to find the cause so that it can be treated. Often once the underlying disease is treated, the hair loss will subside.

Trauma

Areas of hair which are traumatized can result in hair loss. Hot oil hair treatments or chemicals used in permanents may cause inflammation (swelling) of the hair follicle which can result in scarring and hair loss. Trauma such as cuts, scrapes, or burns can result in permanent hair loss if the underlying follicle is damaged. Surgical excision of the scarred area or hair transplant surgery can be undertaken to correct the cosmetic deformity.

Pulling Hair

Finally, tightly pulling hair can cause hair loss. People who wear pigtails, cornrows, or use tight hair rollers can pull the hair and cause traction alopecia. If the pulling is stopped before scarring of the scalp develops, the hair will grow back normally. However, scarring can cause permanent hair loss.

Suggested Questions to Ask Your Physician

What is causing my hair loss?

While unfortunately the cause of hair loss can not always be identified or may be a natural part of aging, always ask before treating. Even self treating with readily available treatments can worsen hair loss. Consultation with a physician specialized in hair loss is sometimes necessary though a good start is visiting your family physician.

Will treatment help?

After you have figured out what is causing your hair loss, determine if treatment is even necessary or will help. For some causes, hair transplants are not an option. If the cause is medication induced, ask your doctor if another medication will work to treat your condition just as well. Just remember, sometimes the treatment is worse than the disease.

Additional Web References

http://www.nlm.nih.gov/portals/public.html

The public information section of the National Library of Medicine web site, this link provides useful information about hair loss in general and specific types of hair loss. Simply type the search term in the box.

http://familydoctor.org/online/famdocen/home/men/general/081.html

Information provided by the American Academy of Family Physicians on hair loss.

http://www.naaf.org

The National Alopecia Areata Foundation provides information for patients diagnosed with the condition as well as listing of regional support groups.

http://www.niams.nih.gov/Health_Info/Alopecia_Areata/default.asp

Information from the National Institute of Arthritis and Musculoskeletal and Skin Diseases about alopecia areata.

http://www.trich.org

The Trichotillomania Learning Center is a national non-profit organization which provides education and support for people suffering from the disease.

http://emedicine.medscape.com/article/1071566-overview

A more in depth discussion of telogen effluvium on emedicine.com.

Part VI

Testing for Hair Loss

For a trained physician, testing is not always necessary. The diagnosis of androgenic alopecia is generally made on history and physical examination alone. For patients with evidence of metabolic disorders or other physical ailments, additional testing for the underlying disease may be necessary. Autoimmune disease blood testing, thyroid function tests, testosterone and dihydroepiandrosterone sulfate (DHEAS) levels, as well as cancer screenings may be necessary if other parts of the patient's history warrant.

For some patients with a less well defined cause of hair loss, hair loss tests may be in order. The pull test can be used to test for telogen effluvium. Gentle pulling is done on a bunch of hairs in at least 3 different parts of the scalp, with at least one of the areas just above the ear. Less than 6 hairs should be removed at any one spot. If the pull test is equivocal, patients may collect a weeks worth of hair from the shower and comb, count the number of shed hairs, and have the physician examine the hairs. This can help to identify if an abnormal number of hairs are being shed and telogen effluvium is suspected.

The pluck test can be utilized to examine the hair bulb and determine which phase of the hair cycle hairs are in. Several hairs are plucked from the scalp to extract an in tact bulb. The morphology of the bulb can tell the physician the stage of the growth cycle and suggest a cause for the loss.

Scalp biopsy is often necessary when the diagnosis of the hair loss is in question. Biopsy should be performed at the edge of a bald patch and can help to identify infections, some autoimmune diseases, alopecia areata, systemic sclerosis, and neoplasms.

If hair pulling is suspected, a small area of the scalp can be cut short and covered with a dressing. In a week, the patient is asked to return to the office and the area is checked. If normal hair growth is noted, trichotillomania can be suspected.

For patients with androgenic alopecia who are trying alternative treatments to surgery, hair counts with specialized devices can be undertaken to help provide an objective evaluation of the efficacy of the treatment.

Part VII

Categorizing Alopecia

Androgenic alopecia, unlike other types of hair loss, follows a fairly well defined pattern in men. Though women also follow a pattern, it is less well defined and different from the hair loss experienced by men. Several attempts have been made to categorize hair loss but due to the difference between male and female hair loss, two different systems have become the standard for classification: Norwood classification for male pattern baldness and Ludwig classification for female alopecia.

Hamilton, an anatomist, recorded his observations of more than 300 men and graded their patterns of hair loss in 1949. Dr. O'tar Norwood, a dermatologist and distinguished hair transplant surgeon, expanded Hamilton's classification after conducting his own study of 1,000 men. The Norwood classification, published in 1975, is the most widely used classification for hair loss in men. It defines two major patterns and several less common types. As Norwood observed, thinning starts in both temples as well as the crown/vertex and slowly progresses to encompass the entire top of the scalp.

Unfortunately, the hair loss classifications promoted by Hamilton and Norwood do not adequately reflect the hair loss observed in women suffering from alopecia. In 1977 the Ludwig classification of female hair loss was proposed and today is the most widely used classification system for female hair loss in the world.

Scales of both grading systems are provided on the next page.

Norwood Classification for Male Pattern Baldness

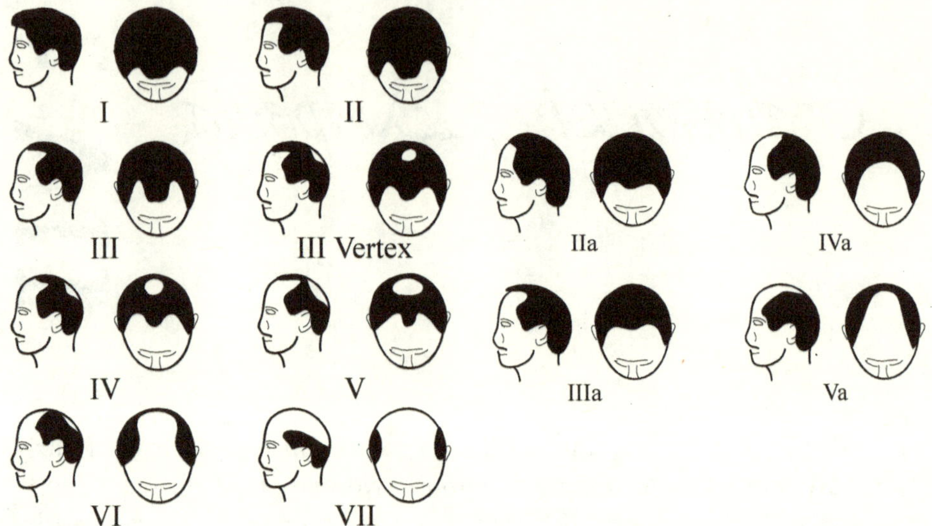

Ludwig Classification for Female Hair Loss

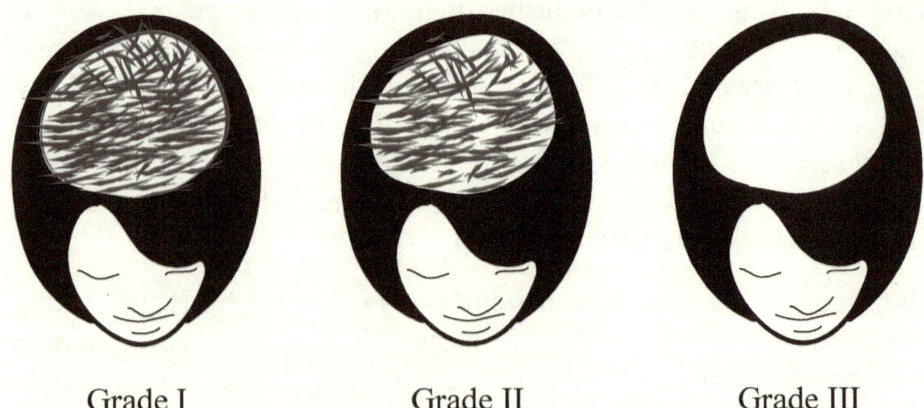

Part VIII

Nutrition

Hair is one of the most metabolically active parts of the body. As such, it takes a lot of nutrients to ensure that it can adequately grow. A balanced diet with appropriate calories, vitamins, and minerals is essential for good overall body health and hair health. Some minerals and compounds cannot be made by the body, therefore exogenous intake is necessary.

Fats

A balance must be obtained with fat intake. While much attention is paid in Western culture to a decrease in fat intake, there are some fats which are good and essential to normal body activity. Fatty acids, such as omega-3 and omega-6 oil, can only be obtained through sources outside of the body and must be consumed for normal body function. The most common natural sources of these 'essential fatty acids' are fish (salmon, sardines, tuna), plant (flaxseed, soybeans, pumpkin seeds), and walnut oils. It is well documented that essential fatty acid deficiency and generalized malnutrition can cause hair dryness, dandruff, change of hair color, and scalp redness. These effects are usually seen after 2-4 months of inadequate fatty acid intake. The condition resolves when adequate essential fatty acids are consumed.

A balance must be struck though as there is suggestion that excess saturated animal fat intake may cause hair loss. This suggestion comes from the observation that male hair loss in the Japanese population has increased since World War II as has the level of saturated animal fat intake. Though a direct correlation has not been established, the observation is interesting and provides further fuel to the controversy over diet and hair loss.

Vitamins

A quality multi vitamin which is gender and age specific is always a good idea – but can be essential for those wishing to slow hair loss. Be careful though – you can have too much of a good thing. Excess of certain vitamins can lead to hair loss. Most people are familiar with the RDA of vitamins, or recommended dietary allowance. This system of suggesting adequate intake of vitamins and minerals has been used since 1941. It is regularly updated and in 1997 underwent an overhaul by the Food and Nutrition Board of the National Academy of Sciences with the creation of the Dietary References Intake (DRI). The DRI provides suggested vitamin and mineral intake for males and females dependent on age and pregnancy status.

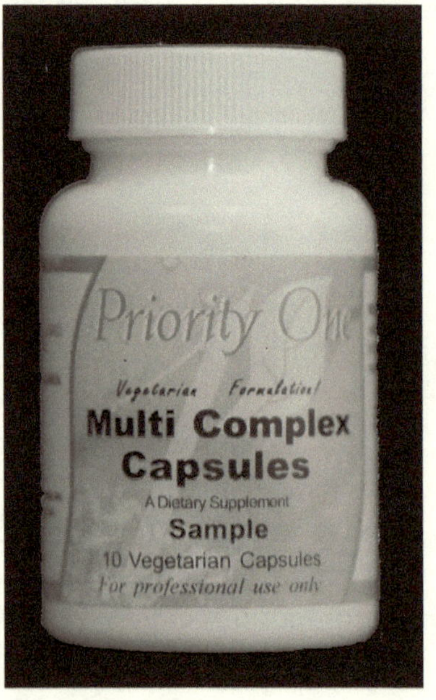

Vitamin A

Vitamin A helps to protect hair follicles from damage by free radicals. A diet low in vitamin A can lead to dry hair. Alternately though, a diet high in vitamin A can lead to hair loss.

The recommended daily intake of vitamin A is 900 μg/d for adult males, 700 μg/d for adult females, 770 μg/d for pregnant adult females, and 1,300 μg/d for lactating adult females. Vitamin A is a fat soluble vitamin meaning that excess intake will be stored in a person's body fat and will not be excreted in the urine. Vitamin A can be derived from liver, dairy products, fish, darkly colored fruits, and leafy vegetables. Beta-carotene can turn into a form of vitamin A. Beta-carotene can be found in carrots, pumpkin, sweet potatoes, winter squashes, cantaloupe, pink grapefruit, apricots, broccoli, spinach, and most dark green, leafy vegetables.

B-complex Vitamins

B-complex vitamins include thiamin, riboflavin, niacin, pyridoxine, cobalmin, biotin, pantothenic acid, and folate. It is believed that the B-complex vitamins contribute to the nourishment of the hair follicle. Deficiencies have been associated with neurologic problems and anemia. B-complex vitamins should be taken as a balanced supplement of all of the vitamins. Natural sources include fortified cereals, organ meats, fortified soy-based meat substitutes, fish, poultry, meat, and some whole grain products. Adequate pantothenic acid intake should be 5mg/d for adult males and females, 6 mg/d for pregnant adult females, and 7 mg/d for lactating adult females. Riboflavin (B2) intake should be 1.3 mg/d for adult males, 1.1 mg/d for adult females, 1.4 mg/d for pregnant adult females, and 1.6 mg/d for lactating adult females. Thiamin (B1) intake should be 1.2 mg/d for adult males, 1.1 mg/d for adult females, 1.4 mg/d for pregnant adult females, and 1.4 mg/d for lactating adult females. Pyridoxine (B6) intake should be 1.3 mg/d for males ages 14-50 and 1.7 mg/ for adult males over 50, 1.3 mg/d for females 19-50 and 1.5 mg/d for females over 50, 1.9 mg/d for pregnant adult females, and 2.0 mg/d for lactating adult females. Finally, cobalamin (B12) should be taken as 2.4 μg/d for adult males, 2.4 μg/d for adult females, 2.6 μg/d for pregnant adult females, and 2.8 μg/d for lactating adult females.

Additional information is available about folate and biotin. Biotin, also referred to as vitamin H or B7, is a water soluble part of the B-complex of vitamins. It is required for cell growth, the production of fatty acids, and the metabolism of amino acids. In a 2000 study, researchers from Harvard University suggest biotin is one of the most important nutrients for preserving hair strength, texture and function. It is found in beans, bread, fish, and legumes. Deficiency is rare but can result in hair loss including eyebrows and eyelashes. Adequate intake of biotin is 30 μg/d adult males, 30 μg/d for adult females, 30 μg/d for pregnant adult females, and 35 μg/d for lactating adult females. Excessive consumption of raw eggs, which contain the protein avidin, can result in biotin deficiency as avidin binds biotin and makes it unavailable to the body.

Folic acid is very important for cell division and multiplication in the body. Signs of folic acid deficiency include anemia, increased fatigue, and graying of hair. Certain medications, especially methotrexate, can lead to folic acid deficiency. There is also good evidence to show a decrease in people exposed to ultraviolet radiation, the same radiation seen in tanning beds and sun exposure. Folate consumption should be 400 μg/d for adult males and females, 400 μg/d for pregnant adult females, and 500 μg/d for lactating adult females. Women who are pregnant or trying to become pregnant should consult with their doctor as birth defects have resulted from folic acid deficiency and additional intake may be necessary.

Vitamin C

Vitamin C helps to protect cells from damage as a strong antioxidant and is an important part of the pathway which produces collagen, a major component of the connective tissue of the skin and hair follicle. Vitamin C can be obtained from citrus fruits, tomatoes, tomato juice, potatoes, brussel sprouts, cauliflower, broccoli, strawberries, cabbage, and spinach. The recommended daily intake of vitamin C is 90 mg/d for adult males, 75 mg/d for adult females, 85 mg/d for pregnant adult females, and 120 mg/d for lactating adult females.

Deficiency of vitamin C is rare in industrialized countries but manifests as the disease scurvy which was common in the fairly recent past. The disease results from improper collagen formation and manifests in the scalp as bleeding at the base of hair and distinctive corkscrew hairs.

Vitamin E

Vitamin E is actually a series of eight fat soluble vitamins, called tocopherols and tocotrienols, that have antioxidant properties. Vitamin E works with selenium to prevent oxidative damage to cell walls. The body preferentially uptakes alpha-tocopherol. Vitamin E can be found in wheat germ, corn, nuts, seeds, olives, spinach and other green leafy vegetables, asparagus, and vegetable oils (corn, sunflower, soybean, and cottonseed). The daily recommended intake of vitamin E is 15 mg/d for an adult male, 15 mg/d for an adult female, 15 mg/d for a pregnant adult female, and 19 mg/d for a lactating adult female. Based on studies, the American Heart Association in 2004 stated that taking more than 400 IU per day of vitamin E can increase the risk of death due to various reasons.

Minerals

Minerals are inorganic compounds which are necessary in maintaining health. Iodine, selenium, zinc, copper, and iron are important for maintaining hair health as well.

Zinc

Zinc is a mineral found in fortified cereals, red meats, and certain seafood. It is essential for cell replication both in the hair follicle and throughout the body. It also helps to stabilize cell membranes and act as an antioxidant. Intake should be 11 mg/d in adult males, 8 mg/d in adult females, 11 mg/d in pregnant adult females, and 12 mg/d in lactating adult females. A British laboratory study in 1988 showed that at least in the lab, a combination of zinc, vitamin B6, and azelaic acid inhibited 5-alpha reductase by 90% in human skin. Unfortunately, further human studies have not been undertaken.

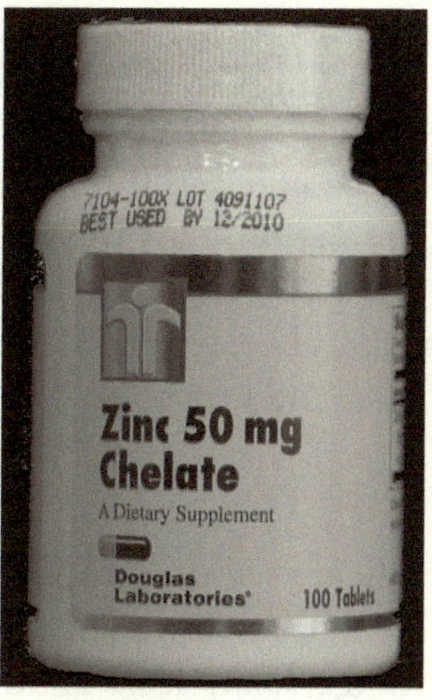

Iodine

Iodine is essential to thyroid function. As mentioned, thyroid dysfunction can manifest as hair abnormalities. Iodine can be found in seafood, some processed foods, and iodized salt. Suggested intake for adult males is 150 μg/d, 150 μg/d for adult females, 220 μg/d for pregnant adult females, and 290 μg/d for lactating adult females.

Selenium

Selenium is necessary for proper iodine useage and proper thyroid function. Selenium deficiency has been shown to result in cancer, heart disease, and poor hair growth. Selenium can be found in organ meats, seafood, and plants grown in soil rich in selenium. Recommended daily intake is 55 μg/d for adult males, 55 μg/d for adult females, 60 μg/d for pregnant adult females, and 70 μg/d for lactating adult females.

Copper

Copper is found in organ meats, seafood, nuts, seeds, wheat bran cereals, whole grain products, and cocoa products. It is required for several enzymes to function properly. Deficiency results in anemia, diarrhea, general weakness, and baldness. Excess intake is also detrimental and can lead to liver damage. Recommended daily intake is 900 μg/d for adult men, 900 μg/d for adult women, 1000 μg/d for pregnant adult females, and 1300 μg/d for lactating adult females.

Calcium

A part of the body's calcium stores acts on the cell membranes of hair to stimulate hair growth. Recommended intake is 1,000 mg/d for men age 19-50 and 1,200 mg/d for men over 50, 1,000 mg/d for women 19-50 and 1,200 mg/d for women over 50, 1,000 for pregnant adult females, and 1,000 mg/d for lactating adult females. Sources of calcium include milk, cheese, yogurt, corn tortillas, calcium-set tofu, Chinese cabbage, kale, and broccoli.

Silica

Silica, or more properly silicon dioxide, is a mineral found in various crystalline forms such as quartz, opal, sand, agate, and certain plant based foods. Though no studies have shown a biological function in humans, it is postulated that silica helps promote scalp circulation because of its high quantities in certain species of horsetail which has been shown to increase scalp circulation. In addition, silica is used in the formation of keratin sulfate which is a component of the hair shaft.

Iron

Iron is an essential component of hemoglobin, the part of the blood which carries oxygen to the body. Iron deficiency results in anemia, brittle hair, and hair loss. Excess iron can also be detrimental leading to heart disease, possibly cancer, increase in free radicals due to hemochromatosis, and destruction of vitamin E. Iron can be found in fruits, vegetables, fortified bread and grain products such as cereal, meat, and poultry. Recommended daily intake of iron is 8mg/d for adult males, 18 mg/d for females age 19-50 and 8mg/d for females 51+, 27 mg/d for adult pregnant females, and 9 mg/d for adult lactating females.

Proteins

Hair loss or negative changes in hair texture are well documented in patients suffering from malnutrition. Fortunately, when proper nutrition is restored, the hair will return to its normal texture and fullness. According to information from the United States Department of Agriculture dietary reference intake tables:

> *"Proteins from animal sources, such as meat, poultry, fish, eggs, milk, cheese, and yogurt, provide all nine indispensable amino acids in adequate amounts, and for this reason are considered "complete proteins". Proteins from plants, legumes, grains, nuts, seeds, and vegetables tend to be deficient in one or more of the indispensable amino acids and are called 'incomplete proteins'. Vegan diets adequate in total protein content can be "complete" by combining sources of incomplete proteins which lack different indispensable amino acids."*

Recommended protein intake for an adult male is 56 g/d, 46 g/d for an adult female, 71 g/d for pregnant adult females, and 71 g/d for lactating adult females.

Proteins are broken down into their constituent amino acids. These are necessary for the body to recreate proteins it needs for proper functioning. Two amino acids are particularly important for hair health because they contain sulfur: methionine and cysteine.

Methionine

Methionine is an essential amino acid, meaning that the body cannot produce it and it must be consumed. To be processed by the body, the L-methionine form should be consumed. Hair requires the sulfur in methionine for healthy connective tissue formation, normal growth, and appearance. The recommended daily intake of methionine and cysteine is 25 mg/g of protein. Patients can suffer from methionine toxicity. In addition, one of the break down products of methionine, homocysteine, can lead to heart disease.

Cysteine

Cysteine can be made by the body and is therefore a non-essential amino acid. Again, the L-cysteine form is the desired form for intake. There is evidence to suggest that sulfur is missing from patient's hair that is being lost. The recommended intake of cysteine and methionine is 25 mg/g protein. Caution should be taken in patients with diabetes as cysteine can block insulin receptors and increase serum sugar concentrations.

Suggested Questions to Ask Your Physician

Will a diet change affect my other medical conditions?

This is a very important question and one that many patients do not ask. Be sure to talk with your doctor if you suffer from other medical conditions before significantly altering your diet.

Are the supplements I am taking worth the money?

Simply going to the local discount store and buying supplements does not mean that those supplements are worth the money you pay for them. Since there is generally no oversight of supplements by any regulatory board, it can be difficult to tell if you are getting the right dosage or even the right form that is taken up by the body.

Additional Web References

http://www.consumerlab.com/

Consumer Lab is an independent testing program for dietary supplements, such as vitamins and herbs. Reports of the efficacy and contents of various supplements is available by subscription.

http://www.naturalstandard.com/

Another independent web site, Natural Standard evaluates different herbal supplements and their effectiveness.

http://www.nutrition.gov

An official web site of the United States Agriculture Department, nutrition.gov is staffed by Registered Dietitians who work at the USDA's National Agricultural Library as Nutrition Information Specialists. The site provides information about nutrition and diet as well as current dietary reference intakes.

Part IX

Herbal & Alternative Medicine

Some patients are concerned about using medications or undergoing surgery and want to know what other alternatives may be available. Civilizations for thousands of years have tried to treat hair loss. Treatments which are presented here are presented as scientifically as possible. It must be remembered that just because an herb or treatment is available without a prescription does not mean that it is safe, without side effects, or does not interfere with other prescriptions a patient may be taking. A lot of these medications are beyond the scope of control of the United States Food and Drug administration and as such do not have significant scientific data to back up claims of use or safety profiles. Because they are outside of the protection of the FDA, many herbal supplements do not have to disclose all of the ingredients, therefore, purity and concentration cannot be guaranteed. Before starting any medication, either orally or topically, patients should discuss it with their physician or pharmacist to determine if there is any evidence for interaction with other medications they are taking or conditions they have.

American Indians

Though extensive research has not been done, some studies indicate that certain herbs may help to prevent hair loss. For many years, various North American Indians have been using hair washes derived from the

Lygodium japonicum and *Yucca* as treatment for hair loss and thinning. Certain tribes also maintained that European shampoos and soaps resulted in premature graying of the hair and dry hair.

Chinese Medicine

Asians have a lower incidence of baldness than Americans. This may be related to diet as Asians have a diet higher in vegetables and herbs. Research has indicated that one of the amino acids prevalent in legumes, L-lysine, inhibits type II 5-alpha reductase, an enzyme important in androgenic alopecia. For the unfortunate Chinese who suffer from hair loss, traditional Chinese medicine offers several treatment options using natural herbs, some of which have been studied.

In traditional Chinese medicine, it is believed that the pattern of hair loss can indicate nutrition deficiencies and even indicate disease of the internal organs. Frontal hair loss indicates excess liquid and fruit intake while hair loss from the top of the head indicates excess animal protein consumption. Should a person suffer from hair loss of the vertex, excess drug and medication intake should be suspected. Excess sugar and drug intake will be reflected in temporal hair loss.

To treat hair loss, Chinese medicine advocates increase intake of roasted sesame seeds (*Sesamium orientale*), *He Shou Wu*, and *Dabao*. While no studies have been performed on sesame seeds, both *He Shou Wu* and *Dabao* have scientific studies for their effect on hair loss. Unfortunately there aren't many studies and further testing is needed to confirm the results indicated in the current studies.

In 1991, a study in the Netherlands was undertaken which compared *Dabao* to placebo for hair restoration. The study was a double blind study with a placebo arm which made it a very good study. At the end of six months, photos taken at the beginning and end of the study were compared for hair growth. Evaluation was made by both the participants and a panel of reviewers. The study involved 373 participants and the final results showed that both groups showed improvement in hair counts and subjective cosmetic appearance, though the *Dabao* group showed a slightly greater hair count (24 hairs average) and a 5% better report of cosmetic satisfaction. The bottom line is that though modest, there was a slightly better result in the *Dabao* group than the placebo.

He Shou Wu, also known as *Fo Ti* or *Polygoni multiflori*, is prescribed by traditional Chinese medicine practitioners to prevent hair from thinning and graying; strengthen the liver, kidneys, bone, and cartilage; work as a blood tonic; work as a mild laxative; treat high blood pressure; and prevent hardening of the arteries. Though used for many years safely in Chinese medicine, in 2006, the British Medicines and Health Care Products Regulatory Agency (MHRA) released a warning about *He Shou Wu* based on several case reports of liver damage after taking the herb. The MHRA advised "Anyone who has previously experienced any liver complaint or any other serious health complaint is advised not to take *Polygonum multiflorum* without speaking to their doctor first."

In 2002, a randomized placebo controlled study was undertaken using both oral pills and a topical lotion containing *He Shou Wu*. The results were evaluated for hair thickness, perceived appearance, hair loss reduction, and new hair growth. Though the number of patients in each group was small, the *He Shou Wu* products showed more favorable results than the placebo group.

Ayurveda

Ayurveda comes from Sanskrit and literally means 'life science.' It is an ancient Hindu system of traditional medicine practiced for over 5,000 years. In Ayurveda, balding or graying of the hair can be caused by stress, emotional trauma, excessive worrying, sudden blood loss, or excessive sexual activity. There are several herbs and other treatments suggested to treat hair loss by Ayurvedic practitioners. To determine appropriate treatment requires determining a person's constitution using profile tests. These test divide a person's constitutional makeup into three categories: pitta, vata, or kapha.

Delicate hair and a tendency toward early graying and baldness affect people with pitta constitutions. In order to combat hair loss, Ayurveda dictates that those with pitta constitutions should consume hair growth foods such as milk, almonds, sesame seeds, and herbs *ashwagandha*, *bala*, and *amalaki*. Veta hair loss involves dry skin, anxiety, insomnia, constipation, and poor digestion. Treatment would include foods such as onion, garlic, sesame, almonds, eggs, and other dairy foods. Kapha individuals tend to have hair which is dark, thick, and wavy; tend towards being overweight; and can be physically weak. Ayurvedic treatment for this type of hair loss consists of cow's milk, ghee, and butter; a nourishing, high-protein diet of lean meat, fish, and ghee; as well as avoidance of fried foods.

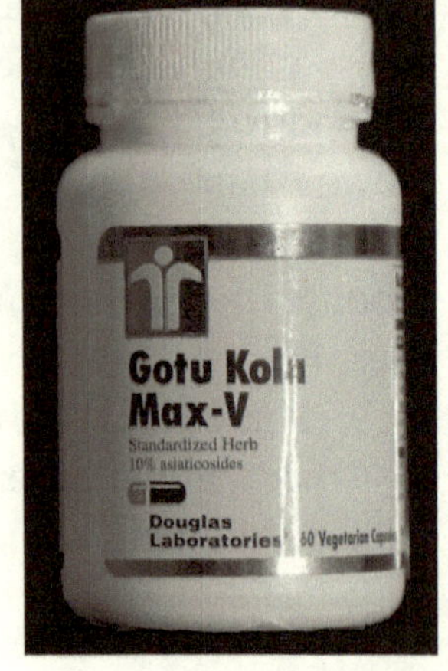

Several herbs are promoted as hair loss treatment by Ayurveda: *gotu kola* (*Centella asiatica*), *bhringaraj* (*Eclipta alba*), *amalaki*, sandalwood (*Santalum album*), and licorice (*Glycyrrhiza glabra*). In a 2008 study, researchers in India studied the effect of topically applied *bhringaraj* extract compared to minoxidil to increase hair growth in rats. The researchers concluded that more hair were in the growth phase in the herbal treatment group than the minoxidil group. In addition to herbs, warmed *bhringaraj* oil and *brahmi* (*Bacopa moniera*) oil should be applied to the scalp on a regular basis. The rice weed plant *Van Bhengra* (*Tridax procumbens*) is used both orally and in hair tonics for hair loss. *Gotu kola*, an important rejuvenative herb in the Ayurvedic teaching is used to treat hair loss as well as to increase nerves and brain cells. No controlled studies have been performed in humans to evaluate their effectiveness at treating hair loss.

In 2007, Indian researchers did look at combinations of three common herbal formulations for hair growth and compared them to minoxidil in shaved rats to determine the time required for complete hair growth. Formulations of *Cuscuta reflexa* (Roxb.), *Citrullus colocynthis* (Schrad.), and *Eclipta alba* (Hassk.) as well as minoxidil were applied topically to the rats. The results indicated increased numbers of growing hairs using the herbal formulations compared to the minoxidil.

Other Herbs

Herbal tea taken both orally and applied to the scalp has been reported to help with hair loss. The most widely studied of the teas is green tea. Some of the compounds in green tea have been demonstrated in the lab and in mice models to increase hair growth with both oral intake and topical administration. It is thought that the compounds work through several methods with one study demonstrating evidence for them to decrease release of 5-alpha reductase genes.

A series of compounds called oligometric proanthocynidin complexes (OPCs) may be useful for hair loss treatment. These compounds can be extracted from the bark of French maritime pine (*Pinus maritime*), grape seeds (*Vitis vinifera*), and apple extracts. OPCs are powerful antioxidants and free radical scavengers. It is thought that they help to support the walls of bloods vessels, decrease inflammation, and improve the support system for collagen and elastin, important components of skin. Based on the results of a lab test in mice, two human trials were undertaken with apple tonic extract applied topically to the scalp. Both studies compared the tonic to placebo and showed an increase in total number of hairs in the treated area over placebo. This suggests that the apple tonic may be useful in hair loss treatment.

Horsetail (*Equisetum arvense*) provides a natural source of selenium, cysteine, and silica – all important in the growth of hair. It is also suggested that horsetail can increase the circulation to the scalp and calcium absorption.

Another herb used to treat hair loss is saw palmetto (*Serenoa repens*). Saw palmetto is a small plum plant which grows in the southeastern United States. Native Americans used the berries to treat urinary retention in older men with difficulty urinating. Several studies have shown the effectiveness of saw palmetto in the treatment of benign prostate hypertrophy (BPH) and lab studies have suggested it may help to treat prostate cancer. While lab evidence in pigs has suggested that saw palmetto works to inhibit 5-alpha reductase, only one study has been done to look at its effect on hair loss. In a controlled study, observers who did not know what medication was given rated that 6 out of 10 of the participants showed improvement in their condition after treatment with saw palmetto. Due to the small size of the study though, definitive conclusions would be difficult to draw and further testing is required.

Care must be taken when taking saw palmetto though. Side effects include mild abdominal pain, diarrhea, nausea and vomiting, and constipation. Men taking saw palmetto have also reported erectile dysfunction, breast tenderness and enlargement, and loss of libido. Saw palmetto should not be taken with other hair loss treatments such as Propecia® as they may adversely affect hormone levels in the body. As with other treatments, it should not be taken by women who are pregnant, thinking of becoming pregnant, or breast feeding as there is no safety data about the product in pregnancy.

Aromatherapy

Societies for centuries have used scalp oil to treat hair loss. Ayurvedic teaching from thousands of years ago includes massaging the scalp with oil. Egyptians believed castor oil could improve hair density and prevent loss. Ancient Indians and Polynesians used coconut oil, and Africans used olive oil to prevent hair loss. Hippocrates, the father of medicine, was even rumored to have applied pigeon dung to his scalp to try to regrow hair. Though not as extreme, recent research shows that scalp oils may be helpful not only with androgenic alopecia but also with alopecia areata.

In a study published in 1998, Scottish researchers looked at daily application of a hair tonic for treatment of alopecia areata. A double blind, controlled study was undertaken with 86 patients. One group massaged essential oils (thyme, rosemary, lavender, and cedarwood) in a mixture of carrier oils (jojoba and grapeseed) into their scalp daily while the other group used only the carrier oils. It was found that 19/43 patients in the treatment group showed improvement compared with 6/41 patients in the control group who showed improvement.

Suggested Questions to Ask Your Physician

Will the herbal supplements interfere with other medications I am taking?

This is a very important question and one that many patients do not ask. Any herbal medication, even though it is sold over the counter, has a risk of interacting with prescription or other over the counter medications. Be sure to discuss with your physician or pharmacist if herbal supplements that you are considering taking will interfere with your other medications - even birth control pills.

Are the herbs I am taking worth the money?

Simply going to the local discount store and buying supplements does not mean that those supplements are worth the money you pay for them. Since there is generally no oversight of herbal supplements by any regulatory board, it can be difficult to tell if you are getting the right dosage or even the right form that is taken up by the body.

Additional Web References

http://www.consumerlab.com/

Consumer Lab is an independent testing program for dietary supplements, such as vitamins and herbs. Reports of the efficacy and contents of various supplements is available by subscription.

http://www.naturalstandard.com/

Another independent web site which evaluates different herbal supplements and their effectiveness.

http://altmedicine.about.com

Information about alternative medicine treatments for various ailments, including hair loss. The articles are not necessarily written by physicians, reviewed, or based on scientific evidence. It does provide additional options for further review.

Part X

Hair Replacement Systems

The practice of wearing artificial hair to cover hair loss dates back centuries. The ancient Egyptians wore wigs to shield their shaved heads from the sun. British royalty wore wigs during the 1600-1700s and wig wearing became synonymous with aristocracy and importance. As a broad category, hair replacement systems can be divided into toupées and wigs. A toupée is a hair replacement system which is small and used to cover a discrete area of bald or thinning hair. Conversely, a wig is a hair replacement system which covers a larger area.

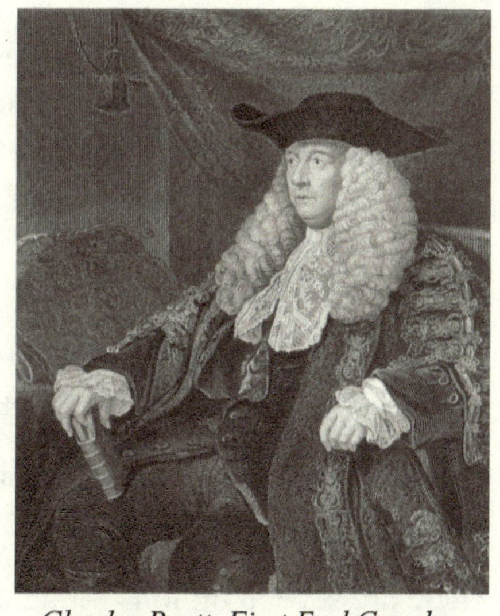

Charles Pratt, First Earl Camden, a British politician who lived in the 1700s sporting his hairpiece.

Hair replacement systems can be a good option for patients because of financial reasons, temporary nature of the hair loss that they are experiencing, and the immediate results which are seen. Hair replacement systems are not without their disadvantages. Patients should be aware of the continued care they must receive and possible significant overall cost before committing to a hair replacement system. Hair replacement systems trap sebum near the scalp which can produce unpleasant odors and possibly accelerate hair loss.

In 1997, Japanese researchers reported a correlation between excess sebum and hair loss. The researchers found that excess sebum can cause high levels of 5-alpha reductase, clog pores, and produce malnutrition of the hair root. By blocking clearing of sebum with a membrane on the scalp, hair systems may inadvertently increase hair loss though no studies have been done to test the hypothesis.

Though hair replacement systems can be a good alternative to more costly hair restoration surgery, patients must remember that quality systems can be very costly, often the same as the more permanent and natural hair restoration surgery. For some patients with extreme hair loss, hair replacement systems may be a better option than hair restoration surgery for a patient's desired density.

Hair replacement systems can be made of human hair or synthetic fiber. The hairs are then tied to some type of mesh base. The bases can be made of several materials including nylon, polyester, silicone, and polyurethane. At times, a combination of materials may be used in the same base to blend better with the skin and create a more natural appearing base. If the mesh is wide enough, the hairs are tied around the mesh itself. For thin mesh, the hair is passed through the mesh and a knot placed on the scalp side of the mesh.

While patients can purchase pre-made hair systems, these will often produce less than desirable results. The most natural appearing systems are those which are custom made of real human hair. Custom systems require the patient to determine the size of the system to be used, the frontal hairline design, the density of the hair, and the color of the hair. Matching density and color to the remaining hair and scalp is critical to ensuring that the hair system appears natural.

Once a hair system has been purchased, attachment and placement are the next steps. If a system is placed incorrectly, it will be detectable. The optimal place for both a hair system hairline and a hair transplant surgery hairline is at the point where the scalp turns from horizontal to vertical.

There are several options for adhering hair systems: glue, tape, or clips. Most systems are secured with either glue or tape and can be applied for one day or up to a month. Before placing the system, the head is thoroughly cleaned and any adhesive left from the previous application is removed. The attachment method is then applied and the hairpiece is placed on the scalp.

Hair systems require routine maintenance. With natural hair, sebum secreted from the scalp coats the hair and helps to keep it maintained. Since there is an artificial layer between the hair and scalp, sebum cannot coat the artificial hair. If the system uses human hair, some sebum will remain on the hair at first but will quickly be removed with wear. In order to keep the system soft and clean, routine cleaning, detangling, and conditioning is required. The system will need to be shampooed but only once or twice a week and blow drying should be avoided. Protection against sun should be used on any hair system to help prevent hair break down through oxidation. Conditioners should be used every day as well after showering.

Hair replacement systems can cost several hundred to several thousand dollars per device. Though they can last for quite some time, they will require replacement, sometimes several times a year. Even with the highest quality system, return to the manufacturer for repair is often necessary on a regular basis. Even the best systems only last 1-2 years. Should the patient experience further hair loss or color change of the hair, new systems may need to be purchased.

Suggested Questions to Ask

What is the cost of the system?

This can get tricky. To determine the cost of the system, determine what each system will cost and if there is any maintenance included in the price. Some companies will require long term contracts to include the cost of maintenance. If so, determine if this includes replacement systems. Before signing any long term contracts, be sure to read the small print.

Who will design my system?

While mail order hair systems can be a good option, the key to a natural look with any hair system is blending of the edges of the hair line with both the natural skin tone and hair color. This can be quite difficult with mail order systems.

What type or hair and base are used?

As mentioned, human hair is the best though most expensive. Bases can vary depending on the desired end result.

Is the hair attached manually or by machine?

Though more operator dependent, manual attachment, when done correctly, will produce a more realistic result.

How often will the system require maintenance?

An excellent vetting question. If the salesperson tells you that their system will never need maintenance, run. Every system requires regular maintenance though timing is dependent on many factors. As a follow up questions, ask what the approximate cost of this maintenance is per year.

How long will the system last?

Again, another excellent vetting question. If you hear that 'n' word again, never, run away. All systems will require replacement at some point though it may be a couple of years.

Is there any warranty?

Inevitably there will be hair breakage and the possibility of more serious damage to the hair system. Determine if there is some type limited warranty to cover hair breakage, damage to the base, or costs associated with poor production.

Additional Web References

http://www.hairdirect.com/

There are many companies which provide hair restoration systems. Hair Direct is one of those companies. I do not recommend one company over another or provide any commentary on their business practices. This web site though has a tremendous amount of patient education about hair restoration systems. There is some bias, obviously, but overall it is an excellent starting point for those who wish to learn more about hair restoration systems.

Part XI

Low Level Laser Therapy

A promising technology for hair growth stimulation which is used in Japan, Australia, and Scandanavia is low level laser therapy (LLLT). LLLT has been used for several decades to treat chronic pain, decrease inflammation, and help with wound healing. There is a large body of evidence to suggest that it helps in these endeavors. Unfortunately, most of the literature to suggest that LLLT helps in hair loss is limited to case reports or studies where no control groups were used for comparison.

The suggestion that LLLT can be used to treat hair loss dates back to the 1960's and a Hungarian researcher named Endre Mester. Mester was the first to use LLLT and was performing experiments in mice to determine if LLLT would be cancerous. He noted that the treated group actually grew hair faster than the non treated group and no cancer formation was noted. Since that time, several LLLT devices have been created. They come in several types but the power of the laser is typically much less than those used for other medical applications.

There is no clear explanation for how LLLT promotes hair growth. One theory is that LLLT somehow increases blood flow to the treated area. Another suggests that LLLT transfers light energy directly to the hair cells and causes increase growth activity through this increase in energy.

It does not appear to work at all on areas which are completely bald and is a treatment that requires constant maintenance to maintain effect.

As noted, there are few placebo controlled, blinded studies to demonstrate that LLLT is effective at treating hair loss. This means that very few studies have compared LLLT to doing nothing. The only study performed to show LLT is better than placebo was one performed by the Lexington International company to gain FDA clearance to market their product called the HairMax Lasercomb® for hair loss treatment. The study showed improvement in density and subjective improvement in appearance for patients using the device over those who used a sham product. Based on this study, the FDA has cleared the company to say that "The HairMax LaserComb® is cleared by the FDA for The Promotion of Hair Growth in males with Androgenetic Alopecia who have Norwood Hamilton Classifications of IIa-V and Fitzpatrick Skin Types I to IV." The study has not yet been published in the medical literature or received review by other physicians prior to publishing.

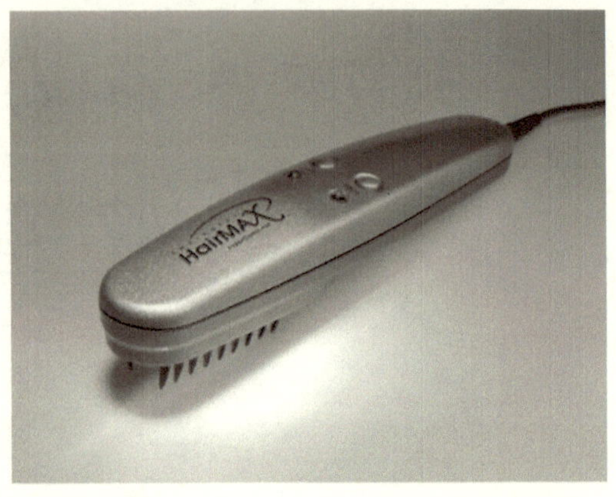

Hairmax Lasercomb®, used with permission of Lexington International LLC

A note here about FDA clearance versus FDA approval. Whenever a product makes a medical claim, such as claiming to treat hair loss, the claim must be evaluated by the FDA. Medical devices are divided into three classes based on their marketed use and potential for harm. The HairMax Lasercomb® is considered a class II device and as such only requires FDA clearance. Clearance is a less stringent standard than approval, which is required for class III devices such as heart stents and other more invasive devices. Clearance only requires that a product demonstrate safety and efficacy compared to similar legally marketed products in the United States. Approval is a stricter standard and requires large studies to demonstrate general safety and efficacy.

There is one independent study performed in 2003 with the HairMax LaserComb® which looked at hair counts and hair tensile strength in 35 patients (28 males and 7 females) over a 6 month period. The authors found an increase in both tensile strength and hair counts in both sexes. Unfortunately there was not a comparison made to doing nothing and the absolute numbers of hairs counted were fairly small.

LLLT appears to be useful for patients both male and female suffering from androgenic alopecia. It does not appear to be effective in treating areas which are already bald and is more effective at treating areas which are thinning. Treatment protocols used in physician offices generally involve treatments 2-3 times per week for 6 weeks then once a week for the next 3-4 months. If positive results are seen, additional touch up procedures are undertaken on a regular basis. Each session takes approximately 20 minutes.

There are two types of LLLT systems available for patients desiring to try it for hair loss treatment. Systems are available which the patient can use at home and larger systems are available for use in physicians' offices. While both laser delivery systems are safe, those used in physicians' offices are stronger and probably deliver a more constant amount of laser energy than the home based systems. The down side is that they are costlier and require repeated trips to the physician's office to have the procedure performed.

There are several devices which are marketed for home use. The HairMax Lasercomb® is the only one which obtained FDA clearance though some of the other devices claim to be FDA approved for hair loss. Office based systems are divided into those which have stationary diodes and those which the diodes rotate around the scalp.

Several words of warning for patients considering LLLT for hair loss treatment. First, be sure to have your hair loss evaluated by a physician before undergoing any type of treatment. For some patients, hair loss is caused by a medical condition which will not respond to LLLT and delay in treatment can cause unnecessary additional permanent hair loss. Second, long term use of the devices has not been studied. The longest studies to date are 6 months long. It is possible that over time, the benefits of the system may not outweigh the cost and time commitment.

Suggested Questions to Ask Your Physician

What is the cost of treatment?

If you are considering LLLT from a physician's office, determine what your cost will be. Remember that touch up procedures are often required to maintain results so determine what the cost of these procedures will be as well as the initial treatment.

Additional Web References

http://www.hairmax.com

The only LLLT device FDA cleared in the United States.

Part XII

Medications for Hair Loss Treatment

There are currently three medications approved by the United States Food and Drug Administration to treat hair loss. Minoxidil and finasteride are approved for hair loss and bimatoprost ophthalmic solution is approved for inadequate or insufficient eyelashes. While some patients may see a perceived increase in hair density after treatment with the medications, they are probably more important in slowing future loss. Patients who undergo hair transplantation are especially urged to begin a regimen of either minoxidil or finasteride to help preserve their current hair density.

Minoxidil

Topical minoxidil, trade name Rogaine® and others, and oral finasteride, trade name Propecia®, are the only treatments for male patterned baldness that have been approved by the US FDA. Their use is indicated in men older than 18 years with mild to moderate hair loss. Several well controlled studies have proven the efficacy of these medications. After 3-6 months of use, slowed hair loss, stabilization, or increased scalp coverage can be appreciated with either medication and results are clearly evident by 1 year. Dense regrowth is uncommon and neither medication can regrow hair in completely bald areas. Early intervention, when thinning is first noticed and hairs are incompletely miniaturized, produces the best results. Treatment must be continued indefinitely to maintain the benefits. Stopping treatment results in a return to pretreatment status by 6 months with minoxidil and by 12 months with finasteride.

For female pattern baldness, 2% topical minoxidil is the only FDA-approved medication. Its use is indicated in women older than 18 years with mild to moderate hair loss. Women who are pregnant or nursing should not use minoxidil.

Rogaine® is distributed over the counter as a 2% liquid or a 5% liquid or foam. There are other formulations of the 2% and 5% liquid sold under various trade names. The foam is only available as Rogaine®. It is recommended to be used twice a day. It is unknown exactly how minoxidil works to slow hair loss. Minoxidil was originally approved to dilate blood vessels and decrease blood pressure. It was noted that increase hair growth was a side effect. This side effect was then used to gain approval for Rogaine®. It is postulated that the increase in blood flow to the scalp caused by dilation of blood vessels somehow causes the increase in hair growth seen with minoxidil.

The most common side effect of minoxidil in its hair loss application is itchy scalp which can be improved by applying only once a day or decreasing medication concentration.

Finasteride

Finasteride for hair loss is only available by prescription and the original tradename was Propecia®. It is a once a day one milligram tablet. The original approval for finasteride was as a five milligram tablet used to treat benign prostatic enlargement. The mechanism of action of finasteride is better understood in hair loss than minoxidil. Finasteride inhibits the activity of type II 5-alpha reductase, an enzyme that converts the male hormone testosterone into a more potent form called dihydrotestosterone (DHT). DHT is believed to act on scalp hair follicles to render them inactive and incapable of producing full-grown hair. By inhibiting the enzyme, finasteride prevents DHT from forming and acting on the hair follicles. Hair loss is then stopped. Unfortunately, the effect is temporary and life long therapy with finasteride is necessary. The most common side effects of finasteride include decrease in libido, erectile dysfunction, male breast enlargement, and depression. When the medication is discontinued, the side effects resolve. Women who are pregnant or may become pregnant should not be exposed to finasteride as it can cause fetal developmental abnormalities. Men who are taking finasteride should advise their physician when undergoing PSA (prostate specific antigen) testing as it can effect the results of the test. This test is commonly performed in older men as a screening for prostate cancer.

According to the Propecia® web site:

> *"PROPECIA was developed to treat mild to moderate male pattern hair loss on the vertex (top of head) and anterior mid-scalp area (middle front of head) in* **MEN ONLY**. *There is not sufficient evidence that PROPECIA works for receding hairlines at the temples.*
>
> *PROPECIA is for the treatment of male pattern hair loss in* **MEN ONLY** *and should* **NOT** *be used by women or children.*
>
> **Women who are or may potentially be pregnant must not use PROPECIA and should not handle crushed or broken PROPECIA tablets because the active ingredient may cause abnormalities of a male baby's sex organs. If a woman who is pregnant comes into contact with the active ingredient in PROPECIA, a doctor should be consulted. PROPECIA tablets are coated and will prevent contact with the active ingredient during normal handling, provided that the tablets are not broken or crushed.**
>
> *In clinical studies for PROPECIA, a small number of men experienced certain sexual side effects, such as less desire for sex, difficulty in achieving an erection, or a decrease in the amount of semen. Each of these side effects occurred in less than 2% of men and went away in men who stopped taking PROPECIA because of them.*
>
> *You may need to take PROPECIA daily for 3 months or more before you see a benefit from taking PROPECIA. If PROPECIA has not worked for you within 12 months, further treatment is unlikely to be of benefit.*
>
> *PROPECIA can only work over the long term if you continue taking it. If you stop taking PROPECIA, you will likely lose any hair you have gained within 12 months of stopping treatment.*
>
> *Although results will vary, generally you will not be able to grow back all the hair you have lost."*

Bimatoprost

Bimatoprost ophthalmic solution is the latest medication approved for hair growth. It was approved in 2009 for inadequate or insufficient eyelashes. The medication is marketed under the trade name Latisse™ and is only available by prescription. The medication was originally approved for treatment of glaucoma. It was noted that a side effect of the medication was eyelash growth. Further studies were done and an indication for eyelash growth was granted by the US FDA. According to the Latisse™ web site:

> *"LATISSE™ solution is intended for* **use on the skin of the upper eyelid margins at the base of the eyelashes. DO NOT APPLY** *to the lower eyelid. If you have a history of abnormal IOP, you should only use LATISSE™ under the close supervision of your physician.*
>
> *LATISSE™ use may cause darkening of the eyelid skin which may be reversible. Although not reported in clinical studies, LATISSE™ use may also cause increased brown pigmentation of the colored part of the eye which is likely to be permanent.*
>
> *You should tell your physician you are using LATISSE™ especially if you have a history of eye pressure problems. You should also tell anyone conducting an eye pressure screening that you are using LATISSE™.*
>
> *The most common side effects after using LATISSE™ solution are an itching sensation in the eyes and/or eye redness. This was reported in approximately 4% of patients. LATISSE™ solution may cause other less common side effects which typically occur on the skin close to where LATISSE™ is applied, or in the eyes. These include skin darkening, eye irritation, dryness of the eyes, and redness of the eyelids."*

Additional Web References

http://www.rogaine.com
http://www.propecia.com
http://www.latisse.com

The official web sites of the first trade names for the three drugs currently approved to treat hair loss in the United States.

Part XIII

Surgical Treatment

Though medical treatments for hair loss have been around for centuries, advances in surgical treatment have only occurred within the last 50 years. The current state of the art in hair transplant technology involves follicular unit grafting. Mention of the progression of technologies is important as some types of hair loss are not amenable to treatment with follicular unit grafting techniques.

Scalp Reduction Surgery

Scalp reduction surgery was a technique initially pioneered to reduce the amount of bald area on the scalp. This alone or in combination with other hair restoration techniques was used to correct hair loss. While the concept is sound, the natural elasticity in the scalp meant that over time, the excised area would relax and the bald area would recur. As a long term solution to hair loss, this did not prove to be a good option.

Classically, one of three different incisions is made to remove skin in cases of diffuse hair loss. In some cases, patients also undergo tissue expansion in the hair bearing area so that larger areas of hair loss could be removed. Tissue expansion involves placing a plastic balloon under the skin which is slowly filled over several weeks with water to cause the overlying skin to grow. Unfortunately, additional hair follicles are not created and as such the expanded area will have a decreased density of hair follicles.

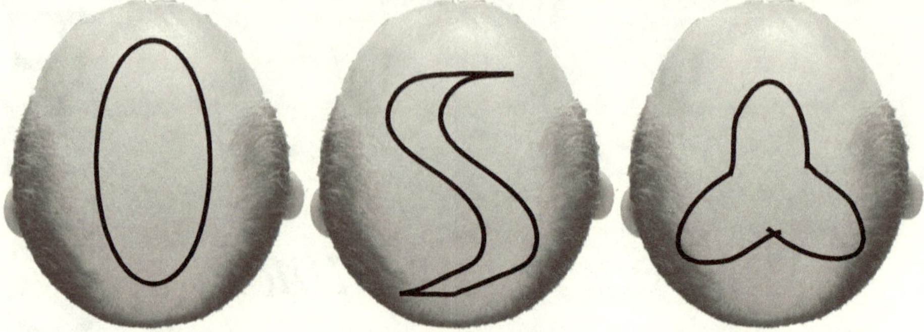

Three common patterns used for scalp reduction surgery.

Scalp reduction surgery runs the risk of scarring, long term recurrence of the bald area, and creation of an unnatural football shaped area of balding as the skin stretches over time. This is termed the vertical slot defect. Several excisions separated by several weeks may be necessary to remove the entire area of hair loss. The resulting hairlines can appear unnatural because of the direction of growth of the hair when it is brought together. Though taught for classical reasons, this technique is not generally used for hair restoration in patients with androgenic alopecia. It is appropriate for patients with small areas of hair loss, for instance due to an accident which caused a scar and bald spot.

Flap Procedures

Though not used for androgenic alopecia, flap procedures are used for patients who suffer full thickness areas of hair loss such as after cancer removal or trauma. Flap procedures are those which take hair and the underlying skin and tissue from one area of the scalp and move it to another area of scalp. The temporoparietal-occipital, or Juri, flap was once used for patients who had androgenic alopecia. The procedure took a strip of hair and skin from the side and back of the scalp and moved it to recreate the frontal hair line. The process took three operations separated by several weeks each.

Complications from the Juri flap included swelling, bruising, and cosmetic imperfections of both the donor and recipient areas. Poor hairline creation because of misdirected hair follicles was common. The flap was also technically challenging for the surgeon and was difficult to obtain reproducible results. It has been mostly abandoned for patients with androgenic alopecia.

In patients undergoing reconstruction of the scalp after trauma or cancer removal, flaps may be necessary to provide the appropriate depth of tissue and blood supple for hair growth. While not a good option anymore for classic androgenic alopecia, scalp flaps are often used in these other situations.

Punch Grafting

The next evolution in hair restoration surgery involved punch grafting. In this technique, a 4mm round punch was used to harvest donor hair from the back and sides of the hair. These grafts contained 4-20 individual follicles with surrounding tissue. The same size punch was used to make recipient sites in the bald area of the scalp. Since the donor hairs do not have DHT receptors, when transplanted, they will not be susceptible to the natural androgenic alopecia progression. The vast majority of the hair would survive and create a lasting head of hair with the patient's own hair. Unfortunately, this technique produced an unnatural appearance to the hair line, often referred to as a doll's head as the hair appeared as the hair on the head of a doll. Though the hair would grow as if it were in its original position, the appearance was less than optimal.

Follicular Unit Hair Transplantation

The early punch grafting has evolved to the current gold standard in hair restoration for androgenic alopecia, follicular unit grafting. In follicular unit grafting, a strip of hair is removed from the back of the head. This strip is usually one to two centimeters wide. The length will depend on the number of hairs required for transplantation and the density of the donor site. The excision can extend from ear to ear along the back part of the scalp. The donor strip is then closed and all that remains is a straight line scar generally well hidden under the hair. Once the strip of hair is harvested, individual follicles are dissected under magnification with either microscopes or special glasses. The resulting graft may contain one to six follicles depending on the surgeon's preference and location of implantation. Once the grafts are created, small incisions are made in the recipient area using specialized knife blades. Using small forceps, the individual hairs are then placed into the recipient sites. The entire procedure can be performed using local anesthesia in an office setting.

Patient Selection

Ideal candidates for follicular unit transplantation have minimal contrast between hair and the background skin, have enough donor hair, are realistic about their results, and are old enough to be able to project future balding. For Caucasian patients, the best transplant candidates are those with gray hair.

Unfortunately there is only a limited donor area for hair. After this donor area is used, no further transplants can be undertaken. Working with a limited resource makes it vitally important to consult with an experienced and trained hair transplant surgeon before undergoing any transplant procedure.

Age is an important factor in hair transplantation. Age and degree of hair loss can give a surgeon some idea of how much hair loss may progress over time. For an older patient with a long history of stable hair loss, additional loss is not expected. For a younger patient with a slowly progressive hair loss, additional loss is the norm. When performing a transplant it must be remembered that the native hair can still fall out with time though the transplanted hair will remain permanently. If a younger person has just the crown area transplanted, they can expect that with time the frontal hairline will recede. This will create an unnatural appearance as the crown and frontal hairline are expected to recede together and will necessitate further surgery to correct the abnormality.

Procedure Preparation

Preparing for a hair restoration procedure starts with education. Learning everything a patient can about the procedure and what to expect is the first step to ensure realistic expectations for results. The next step is the consultation. As explained in both the Choosing a Physician and Advertising Pitfalls sections, consultation should be undertaken with a physician. During the consultation, patients should discuss any other medical conditions they may have with their physician. There are few conditions which make hair transplant impossible but a qualified physician can determine if medical clearance is required before undergoing the procedure. To minimize the amount of bleeding during the procedure and bruising after the procedure, patients should avoid medications that increase the tendency to bleed. Some medications will need to be stopped 1-2 weeks before the procedure. Patients must discuss these with their physician as some medications, especially prescription medications can run significant life threatening risks if stopped. A partial list of over the counter medications which lead to increased bleeding can be found at the end of this chapter. The most common prescription medications which increase the chance of bleeding include coumadin, and Plavix® (clopidegril).

Once you have your consultation and chosen a physician, then it is time for the procedure. Most procedures are performed in a physician's office with local anesthesia or minimal sedation. For the most part, patients are awake for the procedure with minimal discomfort. For most cases, patients should eat a small breakfast and be prepared to have a light snack or lunch during the procedure. Be sure not to dehydrate as longer sessions can last 6 hours or longer and dehydration is a concern. Patients who have only local anesthesia can drive themselves to and from the procedure though a driver is always a good idea, even with local anesthesia. If a patient is not comfortable with only local anesthesia, the consultation is the time to discuss this with the physician as other anesthesia options are available for patients who are anxious.

Design

Well placed grafts will result in a natural appearing hairline. Transplanted hair must not only approximate the outline of the natural hairline, but it must also approximate the angle of the natural hair. When making the recipient sites, a surgeon must be aware of the angle of the hair with the scalp and direction of the natural hair and how it changes over portions of the scalp. For instance, at the front of the scalp, hair is angled forward, while in the temple and sideburns it is angled down. The number of follicles per graft placed in the recipient site is also important to maintain a naturally appearing hairline. Individual follicles placed in a random pattern are used to define the edge of the hairline. Slightly back from the edge, 2-3 follicle grafts are used for added coverage. Beyond this, 1-5 follicle grafts may be safely used to increase hair density and cover a balding area.

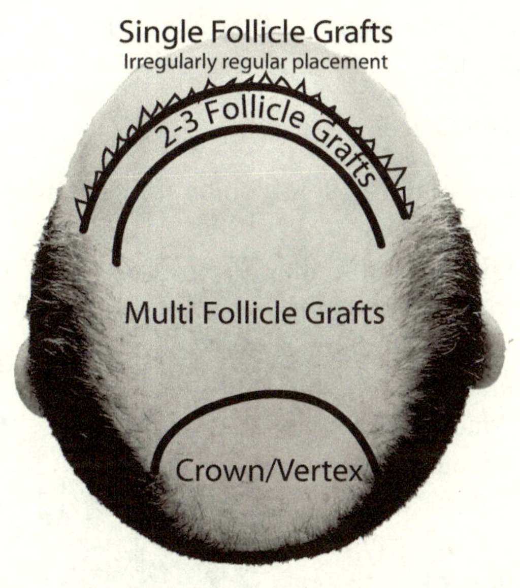

Recreation of a bald crown of the head is a bit more challenging. The crown of the head has significant variation in the angle of the hair. The surgeon must be keenly aware of the varying angulation of this area when recreating the hairline or an unnatural appearance will most certainly result. Most grafts placed in this area are single are at most 2-3 follicle grafts.

For adding density at the top of the head, small squares are created to ensure even distribution of the transplanted hairs. The size and density of each square will depend on a patient's remaining hair density, the number of grafts to be transplanted in the current session, and the size of the area of concern.

In one session of a follicular unit transplant, 500 to 3,000 or more grafts may be placed. Alternately, several sessions may be necessary to obtain the desired result. While one large session can be performed in cases of severe hair loss, multiple smaller sessions may be preferred. Research indicates that graft survival decreases with increasing time out of the body. Larger sessions will necessarily require more time out of the body for grafts and therefore decrease survival. In addition, patients must remember that the donor site is a non-renewable resource – once it is used, it is gone. Should a disastrous outcome or complication occur and a significant part of the donor is used with one megasession there may be little to none left to repair the damage.

The Procedure

For traditional follicular unit grafting with donor strip removal, the procedure is fairly straight forward. Using local numbing medicine, the donor area is injected. The donor area can extend from the top of one ear to the top of the other around the back of the head.

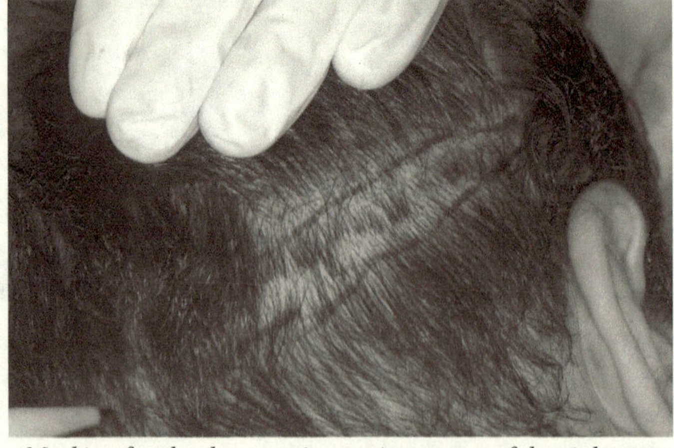

Marking for the donor strip starting on top of the right ear.

It is usually 1-2 centimeters wide. The width and length of the donor area will depend on the number of grafts needed, the density of the donor site, and the laxity of the scalp. For patients with a previous hair transplant and scar from a previous donor site, the scar is incorporated into the new donor site so that the end result is only one scar. The donor site is then harvested down to the fat under the skin. The edges of the wound are brought together and the skin is closed with either staples or sutures.

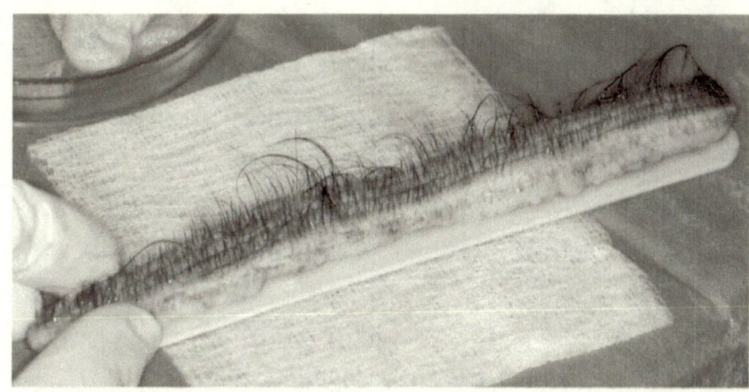

Donor strip after being removed from the scalp.

The key to closure is ensuring that there is minimal tension on the wound edges. Some have described techniques of beveling the edges to allow for hair growth through the incision line. While this can be appealing, even with beveling the edges of the incision, if there is tension on the wound the scar will widen over time. The sutures or staples placed may require removal in 10-14 days or may be allowed to dissolve on their own.

Once the donor strip is harvested, it is passed off to be dissected by the hair technicians. Individual grafts are created. Depending on the hairline design required, single or multiple unit grafts are created.

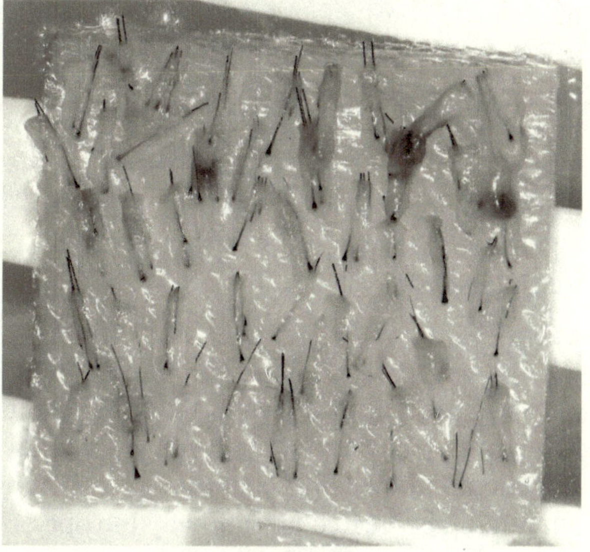

Follicular grafts after being dissected from the donor strip ready for transplant.

After closure of the donor site, patients can usually take a break. At some point just before dissection of the donor tissue is complete,

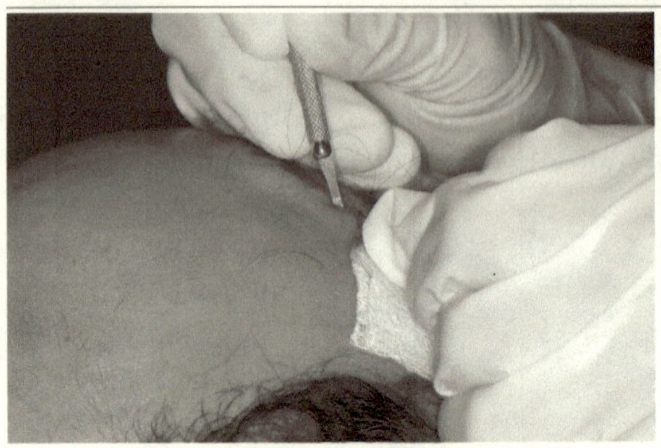

Creation of the recipient sites with special care in angling the blade during insertion.

making incisions at the recipient sites is undertaken. If the area to be implanted is at the front of the hairline, regional anesthesia of the forehead can be undertaken by numbing the major nerves which feed the forehead and frontal part of the scalp. Once the area to be transplanted is numb, small stab incision are made with specially designed knives. Even after initial design and drawings are done, the angle of the blade while making incisions is crucial to ensure that the transplanted hair will grow in a naturally appearing direction.

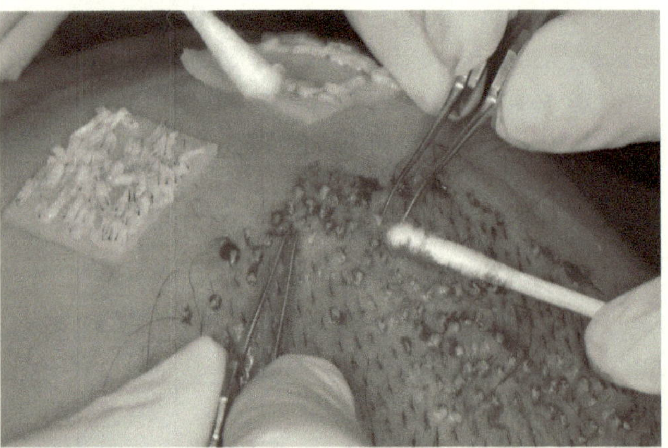

Implantation of the grafts using fine forceps and cotton tipped applicators.

The dissected hairs are then implanted, often using magnification and specially designed forceps to ensure that the hair follicle is not damaged during transplantation.

Risks

The biggest risk of a transplant is the grafts not taking. Overall graft survival has been rated at better than ninety percent in most studies. Infection and bleeding is always possible after any surgical procedure and should be treated promptly by the operating surgeon. Patients prone to abnormal scarring should discuss this with their surgeon in advance as donor site scarring can occur. Keloid formation at the donor site is possible, especially in at risk groups such as African Americans. For scalps which are closed with excess tension, it is possible for the donor site scar to widen over time. This may produce an unsightly scar which can be revised several months after surgery.

Swelling can occur and is variable. If frontal transplants are undertaken, the swelling may descend over the forehead and into the eyes over the next several days after a transplant is performed. This is normal and will subside on its own without compromising the final result.

Patients can expect to have a few in grown hairs which occur as the newly transplanted follicles start to grow. Simply opening the skin over the hair follicle will solve this problem.

Post Operative Course

After the procedure, patients may be asked to wear a headband type of dressing. Instructions for care and return to activities such as hair washing will vary between physicians. Because the transplants are small, the recipient sites heal without being perceptible. A small scab will form over most of the recipient sites and can take a week or longer to resolve. The recipient site will also be red for several weeks. As a natural course after the procedure, most if not all of the transplanted hair shafts will fall out. The follicle remains under the skin but the part of the hair that is seen is shed. It can take several months for the hair to start growing and results are not generally appreciated for three to six months after transplant.

While each physician will have his own postoperative care instructions, I have included a copy of the instructions I provide to patients as a reference at the end of this chapter. It is always crucial to follow the instructions provided by the patient's physician as after care is often as important as the procedure itself in determining final results.

Follicular Unit Extraction

In an effort to provide differentiation, some surgeons have begun harvesting the donor sites through a process termed follicular unit extraction. In a manner similar to previous hair plug removal, very small punches are used to remove single or double follicular unit grafts. The grafts are then transplanted similar to a traditional donor strip follicular unit grafting procedure.

The biggest advantage to this procedure is the lack of a linear scar compared to strip harvesting techniques. For patients who may one day decide to shave their heads, this can be advantageous. Because individual hairs are harvested by one person, operating times for this method are longer than strip harvesting and often more costly. Studies have shown a slightly higher follicular transection rate than with traditional strip donor site harvesting. Unfortunately no clinical studies have been done to compare the results of FUE to traditional donor site harvesting methods. Overall, a clear advantage of FUE to donor strip harvesting has not been shown to make it the preferred method for harvesting donor hair during follicular unit grafting procedures.

Other Donor Sites

For patients with a lack of hair on the head, hair can be taken from the chest, arms, or legs. This is not the ideal donor site as these hairs have different times in each stage of the hair cycle than scalp hair. The biggest difference is a decreased time in the anagen or growth phase resulting in shorter hair than natural scalp hair. This can produce an unnatural hairline or hair appearance.

Other Recipient Sites

Though the scalp is the most common recipient site for follicular unit grafting, other areas of the body can be transplanted as well. Follicular unit grafting can be undertaken for eyebrows, eyelashes, the beard area, and chest hair. The procedure is similar to that which is undertaken for scalp hair transplants. A word of caution though, transplanted hair will continue to grow just as if it were in its original location. If the donor site is the scalp, hair transplanted to other areas of the body may need to be cut on a regular basis to keep it the correct length.

Repair of Previous Transplants

Unfortunately there are patients who have undergone older techniques of hair restoration who have undesirable results. Fortunately, repair techniques have been developed to correct the aesthetics of previous hair plug surgery. By removing some of the plugs and then using those plugs as grafts for follicular unit grafting, surgeons can create a natural hairline where the doll look once existed.

Hair Restoration Instructions

What Can I Expect After Surgery?

There will be a mild to moderate amount of pain and discomfort associated with the surgery. This should be easily controlled with oral medications. Tylenol with codeine (or equivalent if allergy to codeine exists) is generally sufficient for pain control. The discomfort should begin to decrease within 48 hours after surgery and a significant increase in pain after this period should prompt you to call the office.

After surgery, you will have no dressings or bandages on your head. Bring a baseball type cap to wear when you leave the office.

The new hair growth will not start for 4 to 6 months. Prior to this the stubble will fall out and the grafts will look bare. This is completely normal so please do not be concerned. Most of all, be patient during the healing process. The outcome will be well worth the wait.

It is of utmost importance to tell Dr. Verret ahead of time if you have ever been on Accutane, received radiation therapy to the head or neck, or taken steroids or immunosuppressive agents. Immunosuppressed patients (HIV positive, chemotherapy, diabetes, etc.) and patients with certain autoimmune disorders may not be good candidates for this procedure as the risks of poor healing and infection leading to permanent scarring and poor esthetic results may be much higher. It is mandatory that you inform Dr. Verret if you have any of these conditions before surgery.

Things To Remember

- You may drive yourself home after the procedure. It is extremely rare that a patient needs or wants sedation during the procedure(less than 5%). If however, you do need or want sedation, someone will need to drive you home.
- Arrive for your surgery in loose, comfortable clothing. Your top should button or zip rather than pull over your head.
- Be sure to fill your prescriptions before your surgery since it means one less thing for you to worry about afterwards. Take the vitamins and antibiotics until your supply is exhausted; the prescriptions need not be refilled.
- If you are a smoker, you should not smoke for at least 2 weeks prior to surgery and 2 weeks after surgery. Smoking and chewing tobacco inhibit your circulation and can significantly compromise your surgical outcome.
- Do not take any aspirin or any anti-inflammatory compounds for 2 weeks before and 2 weeks after your surgery unless you first discuss it with your surgeon.
- Avoid alcoholic beverages for 48 hours before and 48 hours after the procedure.

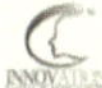

Dr. D.J. Verret ▪ 6545 Preston Road ▪ Suite 200
Plano ▪ Texas ▪ 75024 ▪ phone 972.608.0100

- Wash hair and scalp thoroughly using soap or shampoo on the morning of your procedure. ***Do not*** apply any hair preparation after shampooing.
- Have something light to eat before coming to the office.
- Bring a baseball style cap to wear after surgery.
- Usually you may return to work on the day following your surgery.
- Avoid bending or lifting heavy things for one week. Besides aggravating swelling, this may raise your blood pressure and start bleeding. No lifting over 5 pounds the first week, 25 pounds the second week. After two weeks you may return to all normal activities.
- Avoid straining at stool, which also raises your blood pressure. If you feel you need a laxative, consult your local pharmacist as most stool softeners do not require a prescription.
- Leave the transplanted area open to the air as much as possible. If you plan to wear a hairpiece afterwards, let us know.
- Avoid excessive or prolonged sun exposure to the transplanted area for two weeks. When in the sun, avoid sunburn and use a #15 or higher sunscreen.
- Take only prescribed medication or Tylenol, never aspirin or other NSAIDS, as they promote bleeding.
- On the first night, you may notice a small amount of bleeding at the donor site or the recipient site. This is perfectly normal. To minimize any oozing at the donor site, it is helpful to lie on this area with a towel over your pillow for 2-3 hours when you get home. At the recipient site, just apply pressure with a gauze pad on any small area that is oozing. Significant postoperative bleeding is very rare, but if you suspect it, please call us.
- You may experience some temporary numbness at the donor site. This is completely normal.
- Sleep on your back with your head elevated using a recliner or several pillows for one night after surgery. Do not sleep with head or face in a down position for at least three days.
- The sides and the back of the scalp (including the donor area) may be gently shampooed the first day after surgery and every day thereafter. On the second day after surgery, a light tap water spray can run over the transplanted area. You may decrease the force of the shower spray by crisscrossing your fingers above the transplanted area. Beginning with the fourth day after surgery, you can shampoo the transplanted area just like the back and sides of the scalp. Use your fingertips to gently rub the shampoo in the transplanted area.
- A blow dryer is recommended to dry the hair. This will prevent rubbing the grafts with a towel. The sides and back can be rubbed with a towel. Be sure the setting of the dryer is on warm or cool for the first ten days. Care must be taken as you may have some numbness of your scalp which can cause a burn if the dryer is too hot. Putting your hand where the dryer is focused can prevent developing a burn.
- Sutures used to close the donor site should be removed in 10-14 days. If you live out of town, we can help you arrange for this to be done. At times, we can use dissolvable sutures which will fall out in 2-3 weeks but do not need to be removed. There is no need to be anxious about suture removal – it does not hurt.

DR. D.J. VERRET ▪ 6545 PRESTON ROAD ▪ SUITE 200
PLANO ▪ TEXAS ▪ 75024 ▪ PHONE 972.608.0100

- You can comb your hair the next day, just be careful not to scrape or brush the comb over the grafts. The donor area in the back can be combed immediately, but again, be careful not to catch the comb in the sutures.
- Don't go swimming, diving, or water skiing for at least one month after surgery.
- Do not apply hair coloring until three weeks have elapsed following your operation.
- In 7 - 10 days, the tiny crusts will fall off. Do not pick them. You can speed up this process by putting hydrogen peroxide in a spray bottle and spraying the grafts starting on the fifth day after surgery. Leave the hydrogen peroxide on for 5 minutes, then get in the shower and rinse it off.
- Infection is rare and when it does occur, it is usually very minor. Occasionally a graft will become red, swollen, and tender like a pimple. A topical antibiotic ointment, such as Polysporin (which can be purchased without a prescription), will usually take care of this. Let us know if this does not quickly resolve. An infected graft is a skin problem and does not mean the hair follicles will fail to grow.

Contact the Office Immediately

If you notice any of the following, please contact the office immediately at 972-608-0100:

- unusual bleeding or discharge from the incision.
- development of a temperature elevation exceeding 100.0 degrees.
- a significant progressive increase in pain which is not easily relieved by taking your prescribed medication.

If any of the above should occur after regular office hours, do not hesitate to call Dr. Verret at home at the number provided on the day of surgery or on his cell phone. For whatever reason, if you notice one of the above changes and cannot reach us at our office or through any of the alternate means, present yourself to the emergency department for evaluation.

Recovery Timetable

- **Day 1** Return Home. Take it easy.
- **Days 2** Return to work. Light activities
- **Days 10-14** Remove suture. Return to normal activity.
- **Months 1-4** Transplanted hair may fall out, new hair starts to grow.
- **Months 4-6** Results start to show. Enjoy your new hair.

Remember

If you have any questions at any time, do not hesitate to call. On the day of surgery, you will be provided with Dr. Verret's home and cellular phone numbers as well as the personal contact phone numbers of members of our staff. We do not like surprises and would much rather hear about a small annoyance before it becomes a big problem.

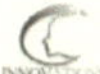

DR. D.J. VERRET ▪ 6545 PRESTON ROAD ▪ SUITE 200
PLANO ▪ TEXAS ▪ 75024 ▪ PHONE 972.608.0100

Over the Counter Medications to Avoid

Certain over the counter medications can effect the ability of the body to form blood clots and stop bleeding. The following list is some of over the counter medications which are known to cause an increase in bleeding tendencies and should be ***avoided two weeks before and two weeks after surgery***. This is *not* a comprehensive list as most over the counter medications have not been tested for their effects on bleeding or photosensitivity. If you have any questions about medications you are taking, please talk with Dr. Verret. In the end, it is safer to avoid the medication if at all possible for ***two weeks before and two weeks after surgery***. Please talk with Dr. Verret about any prescription medications you are taking before discontinuing them.

Aches-N-Pain
Advil
Aleve
Alka Seltzer Effervescent Pain Reliever & Antacid
Alka Seltzer Plus Cold Medicine
Anacin Analgesic Tablets & Capsules
Anacin Maximum Strength Capsules
Anacin Maximum Strength Analgesic Tablet
Arthritis Bayer Timed Release Aspirin
Arthritis Pain Formula
Arthritis Strength Bufferin
Asian ginseng
Ascriptin
Aspergum
Aspirin
Aspirin Suppositories
Bayer Aspirin
Bayer Children's Chewable Aspirin
Bayer Children's Cold Tablets
BC Tablets
Bilberry
Black cohosh rhizome
Black currant
Bladderwrack
Bromelain
Bufferin
Cama Arthritis Pain Reliever
Cama Inlay
Carpon
Cayenne fruit
Celery plant
Children's Advil
Children's Motrin (Ibuprofen)
Chinese skullcap root
Clinoril
Colrex
Congesprin
Coricidin CD
Coricidin Demilets Tablets for Children
Coricidin Medilets for Children
Coricidin Tablets
Coragesic
Da huang
Dan shen root
Decajen
Devil's claw
Diclofenac
Diflunisal
Dolobid
Dong qual
Dristan
Duradyne
Dynasol
Echinacea
Easprin
Ecotrin Tablets
Ecotrin Maximum Strength Tablets
Empirin
EnTab 650
Ephedra
Etodolac
Evening primrose seed oil
Excedrin

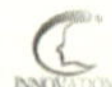

Dr. D.J. Verret ▪ 6545 Preston Road ▪ Suite 200
Plano ▪ Texas ▪ 75024 ▪ phone 972.608.0100

- Extra-Strength Bufferin Capsules & Tablets
- Feverfew
- Fish Oil
- 4-Way Cold Tablets
- Garlic
- German chamomile
- Ginger
- Gingko Biloba
- Ginseng
- Gemnisyn
- Goody's Powder
- Halfprin
- Haltran
- Horse chestnut
- Ibuprofen
- Indocin
- Indomethacin
- IPAC
- Kava
- Lanorinal
- Licorice
- Lodine
- Magnaprin
- Meadowsweet
- Medipren
- Meptogesic
- Midol
- Mobigesic
- Momentum
- Mortin IB
- Naprosyn
- Naproxen
- Norwich Aspirin & Extra Strength Aspirin
- Nuprin
- Onion
- Orudis/Ketoprofen
- PAC
- Pamprin IB
- Pan PAC
- Panax ginseng
- Papain
- Papaya
- Pasibar
- Persistin
- Phenergran
- Phenotron
- Poplar
- Presalin
- Quiet World
- Red clover
- Reishi fruit bodies
- Rindecon
- Rhinogesic
- Ru-Tuss
- St. John's Wort
- St. Joseph Aspirin for Children
- St. Joseph Cold Tablets for Children
- Sine-Off Sinus Medicine, tablets, Aspirin
- Sine-Aid
- Sinutab
- Sulindac
- Sweet birch bark
- Sweet clover
- Sweet scented bedstraw plant
- Sweet vernal grass leaves
- Tamarind
- Therapy Bayer
- Tonka bean seeds
- Trendar
- Triaminic Tablets
- Trigesic
- Turmeric root
- Ursinus
- Valerin
- Vanilla leaf leaves
- Vanquish
- Vitamin E
- Voltaren
- Willow bark
- Wintergreen
- Woodruff plan

Remember – Stop using these medications for at least 2 weeks before and 2 weeks after surgery

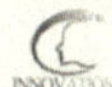
DR. D.J. VERRET ▪ 6545 PRESTON ROAD ▪ SUITE 200
PLANO ▪ TEXAS ▪ 75024 ▪ PHONE 972.608.0100

Suggested Questions to Ask Your Physician

What are my treatment options?

There are always options - even if it is to do nothing. Always ask the physician with whom you consult what all of your options are before proceeding.

How many grafts do you think I will need?

While it is impossible to determine exactly how many grafts a patient will need to get the density that they wish for, most physicians can give a reasonable estimate.

What is your price structure?

Determining price structure is key to comparing transplant surgeons. Some surgeons charge by the session, some by the graft, and some by the hair. If the surgeon charges by the graft, be sure to ask how many follicles he expects per graft. If the surgeon only places single follicle unit grafts, the cost is more comparable to a by the hair cost. Be sure to also ask about how future transplant sessions are charged. Some physicians will charge additional sessions as if they are unrelated to the first while others will consider it a continuation of the first session. Check out the Advertising Pitfalls section for a more in depth discussion of comparing pricing structures.

What are your post operative instructions?

Every physician has different instructions for care after your procedure. Some will require bandages on the scalp for a time period while others may place restrictions on travel or activity. Be sure to talk with your physician about their routine instructions so there are no hard feelings after the procedure.

Additional questions to ask when considering hair restoration procedures are included in the Choosing A Physician section.

Part XIV

Hair "Cloning"

Much attention has been paid recently to a process which is generally termed hair cloning. When performing hair transplants, the biggest limitation to creating a completely natural and full head of hair is the limited donor site. For patients with complete balding, there is not enough donor to recreate a full head of hair like patients had in their teens. But, if a person's hair could be grown in the lab and then transplanted, the solution would be easy. Cloning implies making an exact genetic copy of an organism. Hair is quite a complicated structure, made up of many types of cells and other appendages. Current technology relies on tissue engineering rather than actual cloning of hair.

The search for methods to grow hair dates back to the 1960's. At that time, Roy Oliver, a British researcher, demonstrated that taking a dermal papilla from a growing hair and placing it into a follicle which lost its papilla would result in hair growth. The papilla is the part of the follicle at the base which is responsible for hair growth and response to androgens. Oliver further showed that transplanting an intact papilla could cause a new follicle to grow in skin which had lost its follicles.

Interestingly, in the late 1990's, researchers found that the dermal papilla can be implanted into unrelated persons without being rejected. As it turns out, the papilla lacks the genetic information which identifies tissue as foreign. This means that dermal papilla could be grown in culture and banked for future use in different patients though no research has been performed to date on the topic.

Even with decades of research, hair tissue engineering has not proven a viable option for hair restoration though much research continues to be done. There are several obstacles which must be overcome.

First, identification of the exact cells to be used for the cloning has not been worked out. Would the best clones come from the person, another person, or even another species? What are the best cells to produce the best hair? Once these questions are answered, the next technical obstacle is reliably removing the cells. The cells must be then cultured and replicated outside of the body.

Another major hurdle is creating a medium in which to grow the cells which will reliably create what we identify as hair. At this point, simply replicating the dermal papilla cells does not reliably guarantee growth of a follicle and associated appendages. Even with the medium, guaranteeing that the resulting hair has the proper texture, color, and orientation of growth is another hurdle.

Last, long term studies will have to be done to ensure that implanted cells do not increase the risk of tumor formation. One study performed in 1998 in animals showed no tumor growth with implanted dermal papilla cells suggesting that the technology may be viable.

Outside of the scientific challenges, regulatory hurdles will have to be overcome as well. Given the process of regulatory approval required by the US FDA, it is likely that any viable hair engineering technology will be available oversees before it is available in the United States. Needless to say, the technology is many years from being a viable option for hair restoration.

Additional Web References

http://www.intercytex.com/
http://www.histogeninc.com/
http://www.aderansresearch.com/

These are the corporate web sites for several companies developing hair replacement tissue engineering technologies.

Part XV

Smoking and Healing

A special section needs to be dedicated to the effects of smoking on wound healing. The idea behind cosmetic surgery is to undergo procedures which can improve the way a person look. Unfortunately, smoking can significantly increase a patient's risk of wound healing problems and put you at risk for poor results after your procedure.

Smoking will increase a person's heart rate 10-20 beats/minute and increase blood pressure by 5-10 mm mercury. Any increase in blood pressure and heart rate can increase the risk of bleeding in the post operative period. Increases in blood sugar caused by smoking can cause blood cells to clump together and cause blood clots in the small vessels forming in the healing tissue, blocking necessary oxygen and nutrients. In long time smokers, coughing can persist which increases blood pressure predisposing to bleeding and decreasing the ability of the lungs to exchange carbon dioxide for oxygen.

Individual components of smoke can also be detrimental. Nicotine causes blood vessels to constrict and increases the chance of blood clots. Both of these effects can decrease the ability of oxygen and nutrients to get to the healing areas of the skin. On a microscopic level, nicotine inhibits macrophages and fibroblasts, blood cells necessary for proper wound healing. Even in patches and gum, nicotine can cause problems with wound healing.

Carbon monoxide in smoke combines with hemoglobin, the oxygen carrying compound in the blood, to form carboxyhemoglobin. Carboxyhemoglobin decreases the ability of the blood to carry oxygen to the healing tissues.

Numerous studies have shown an increase risk of wound healing complications including skin death, scarring, and infection in patients who smoke over those that don't. Patients who have a facelift and smoke have a ten times greater risk of death of the skin of the face than those who don't smoke. Studies have suggested that if a patient is able to stop smoking for two weeks before and two weeks after surgery, the risk of complications, though increased over non-smokers, is reasonable and significantly decreased over active smokers.

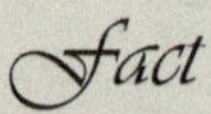

Cotinine testing can determine nicotine use for 4 days before testing.

Cosmetic surgery can provide the incentive for smoking cessation. If a patient is able to stop smoking to have a cosmetic procedure performed, often they will stop smoking permanently.

Part XVI

Choosing a Physician

When choosing a physician for hair loss, there are two aspects to consider - diagnosis and treatment. Physicians who treat hair loss will often be able to diagnose hair loss but sometimes may opt to defer treatment for medical causes to more qualified individuals. Often primary care physicians, such as family physicians, internal medicine physicians, or gynecologists, can diagnose straight forward hair loss. Dermatologists are specially trained in diagnosing and treating diseases of the skin including hair loss and referral to a dermatologist may be necessary in more difficult cases. For hair loss treatment by surgical hair restoration procedures, it is important to choose an experienced and trained physician to get the best results possible.

There is a huge market for hair loss treatments which has spawned many businesses which claim to treat hair loss. Surgical treatment too has several large multinational organizations which provide treatment, sometimes at the cost of personalized care and individual results.

There is no set method to choosing a physician. First and foremost, you must be comfortable with the person to whom you are trusting your face. The rest of the suggestions provided should be taken together as a whole to make your decision. No one factor is more important than another in determining a competent physician. Taken as a whole, they provide a good starting point to get the best results possible.

Board Certification

Board Certification refers to accreditation a physician receives by completing some form of testing to demonstrate competence in a specific field. In the United States, the standards for board certification are administered by the American Board of Medical Specialties (ABMS), a not-for-profit organization. The ABMS is composed of 24 approved medical specialty boards. These boards include:

- allergy and immunology
- anesthesiology
- colon and rectal surgery
- dermatology
- emergency medicine
- family medicine
- internal medicine
- medical genetics
- neurological surgery
- nuclear medicine
- obstetrics and gynecology
- ophthalmology
- orthopaedic surgery
- otolaryngology
- pathology
- pediatrics
- physical medicine and rehabilitation
- plastic surgery
- preventative medicine
- psychiatry and neurology
- radiology
- surgery
- thoracic surgery
- urology

Each board has its own set of criteria to become board certified. Generally these criteria include completion of an MD or DO degree program in the United States or equivalency testing for foreign medical graduates; completion of a board approved training program (often referred to as residency); completion of a written and oral examination; and for some surgical specialties, demonstration of skill competency through a certain period of time in practice or submission of case logs. Each board as well may have specialty areas which provide additional certification through associated boards. Before 2000, board certification was performed once in a physician's career. As of 2006, board certification must be renewed every 10 years though certain physicians have been grandfathered into the lifetime certificates.

Currently, there is ***no*** ABMS member board which certifies hair restoration surgeons. Therefore, consideration is made to a broader category of cosmetic and reconstructive procedure certification. The three boards generally acknowledged to train physicians in cosmetic and reconstructive skin procedures are: The American Board of Dermatology, the American Board of Otolaryngology, and the American Board of Plastic Surgery. According to the ABMS website:

- *"A Dermatologist is trained to diagnose and treat pediatric and adult patients with disorders of the skin, mouth, external genitalia, hair and nails, as well as a number of sexually transmitted diseases. The Dermatologist has had additional training and experience in the diagnosis and treatment of skin cancers, melanomas, moles and other tumors of the skin, the management of contact dermatitis and other allergic and nonallergic skin disorders, and in the recognition of the skin manifestations of systemic (including internal malignancy) and infectious diseases. Dermatologists have special training in dermatopathology and in the surgical techniques used in dermatology. They also have expertise in the management of cosmetic disorders of the skin such as hair loss and scars and the skin changes associated with aging."*

- *"An Otolaryngologist-Head and Neck Surgeon, provides comprehensive medical and surgical care for patients with diseases and disorders that affect the ears, nose and throat, the respiratory and upper alimentary systems, and related structures of the head and neck. The Otolaryngologist diagnoses and provides medical and/or surgical therapy or prevention of diseases, allergies, neoplasms, deformities, disorders and/or injuries of the ears, nose, sinuses, throat, respiratory and upper alimentary systems, face, jaws and the other head and neck systems. Head and neck oncology, facial plastic and reconstructive surgery and the treatment of disorders of hearing and voice are fundamental areas of expertise." Further training can be undertaken to obtain a subspecialty in Plastic surgery Within the Head and Neck.*

- *"A Plastic Surgeon deals with the repair, reconstruction or replacement of physical defects of form or function involving the skin, musculoskeletal system, craniomaxillofacial structures, hand, extremities, breast and trunk and external genitalia or cosmetic enhancement of these areas of the body. Cosmetic surgery is an essential component of plastic surgery. The Plastic Surgeon uses cosmetic surgical principles to both improve overall appearance and to optimize the outcome of reconstructive procedures. The surgeon uses aesthetic surgical principles not only to improve undesirable qualities of normal structures but in all reconstructive procedures as well.*

Special knowledge and skill in the design and surgery of grafts, flaps and free tissue transfer and replantation is necessary. Competence in the management of complex wounds, the use of implantable materials and in tumor surgery is required. Plastic Surgeons have been prominent in the development of innovative techniques such as microvascular and craniomaxillofacial surgery, liposuction and tissue transfer. Anatomy, physiology, pathology and other basic sciences are fundamental to the specialty.

Competency in Plastic Surgery implies an amalgam of basic medical and surgical knowledge, operative judgment, technical expertise, ethical behavior and interpersonal skills to achieve problem resolution and patient satisfaction"

There is no national law which sets forth criteria for what organization can call themselves a board or provide physicians with board certification. Some 'board certification' involves simply paying a fee and receiving a certificate, similar to belonging to a medical society. Should you question the qualifications for a board certification, be sure to visit the board's web site. Reputable national boards will provide the qualifications for certification and identify qualified physicians. At minimum, the certification should include a written examination, verbal examination, and some form of continuing maintenance of certification.

Remember that appropriate board certification ensures that a physician has the minimum competency in his/her field. This does not guarantee results or that a physician has had appropriate training in newer procedures introduced since residency.

Special mention should be made of the American Board of Hair Restoration Surgery (ABHRS). The ABHRS is not a member board of the ABMS but does certify surgeons in hair restoration surgery through experience, written testing, and oral testing. Due to the lack of ABMS membership, lack of oversight by any nationally recognized governing board, and no official medical residency in hair restoration, most states do not recognize 'board certification' from the ABHRS and limit advertising this credential. Because of these limitations, many well qualified physicians do not undertake the added expense of credentialing with the ABHRS.

Training

Ensure that a physician is trained to do what they are doing. If a physician is board certified and the certifying board condones cosmetic and reconstructive procedures, this will ensure a basic training has been undertaken. If a physician is board certified by a board which does not specifically deal with cosmetic and reconstructive concerns, ensure that the physician has gone through additional extensive training in hair restoration surgery. For some this may include additional observation of physicians or extensive training courses. Beware though of physicians who have a certification from a weekend course or some other process to do something which is completely outside of their initial medical training.

Though board certification will ensure the basic training to participate in a particular field of medicine, just completing a residency does not ensure that a physician is trained in the procedures they are performing. Simply asking how many of a procedure a physician has performed also is not completely informative. Adding 2+2 and getting 5 several hundred times does not make it happen. Similarly, just because someone has performed 500 hair transplant procedures, doesn't mean that they perform them well or can adequately address the desires you have for your procedure. Training and experience must be taken together with all of the other criteria before choosing a physician.

Faculty Appointments

Physicians do not have to be employed by a university to have an appointment to the faculty of the university. Often, private practice physicians will volunteer time to teach at medical schools and residency programs. For their time, they may receive an appointment as a clinical faculty to the medical school. These appointments usually do not have any monetary reimbursement associated with them but reflect the physician's commitment to continuing education.

Articles and Presentations

Though the demands of a busy practice can be great, physicians will often publish peer reviewed articles in scientific journals and speak at national and international physician society meetings. There is generally no financial reward for these presentations and journal articles. By writing and presenting, a physician shows commitment to continuing education, illustrates that they have techniques which other physicians are interested in learning, and demonstrates that they have enough patient flow to report results in the medical literature. Peer review indicates that the articles or presentations are reviewed by other physicians in the same field before publishing. In contrast to columns published in mainstream media, a peer reviewed publication requires approval of other physicians before publishing helping to ensure that topical and factual presentations are presented.

Hospital Privileges

Unfortunately all medical procedures have some risks, even hair restoration procedures. Though significant complications with hair restoration procedures are rare, they do occur and hence the need for informed consent. For a physician to practice medicine, hospital privileges are not required. Unfortunately, some complications from hair restoration procedures do require hospitalization and as such, having a physician who can admit you to the hospital can be life saving. If your physician does not have hospital privileges, you may be entrusted to the care of someone who is not familiar with the procedure that you underwent or you may have to be sent to a facility with a higher level of care a distance from your initial physician. Be sure to ask your physician where they have hospital privileges.

Local versus National

The cash nature of the business and large population with hair loss has sprouted a large industry. Many national and international firms employee physicians to perform hair restoration procedures. While some of these physicians are very good at what they do, caution should be taken. Patients should remember that they are often entering into a contract with a large corporation whose focus is on the bottom line and not the hairline. Local physicians with roots in the community will be interested in obtaining good results for a patient, not only for the patient's benefit but to maintain their reputation in the community. Local physicians are more likely to make accommodations for patients when things do not turn out as expected. Most physicians performing cosmetic surgery understand that the surgery is a large investment and only the beginning of the doctor/patient relationship.

Hair Technicians

Not enough can be said about choosing a physician with experienced hair technicians. Follicular unit grafting techniques require dissecting hundreds if not thousands of individual hair follicles. This can not be undertaken by just one person. Technicians are vital to assisting the physician in dissecting the individual follicles and placing them. Ensure that any physician you are considering working with utilize only highly trained and experienced hair technicians. This will decrease the operative time and improve hair survival in the long run. Be sure to ask what part the technician plays in the procedure though. Unless they are appropriately licensed in the state, such as nurses or some surgical technicians, hair technicians should not be performing injections. They should definitely not be left to perform either donor site harvesting or recipient site incisions. These are procedures which should be performed only be the physician.

Some physicians will employ hair technicians full time. Others may opt to contract with certain hair technicians on an as needed basis. There are many hair technicians who fly around the country assisting doctors in transplants but do not work with only one physician. In either case, ensure that your physician is employing hair technicians who are experienced and not simply employing untrained man power to perform the dissections and placement.

Microscope Usage

Much attention has been focussed on microscope usage for hair dissection. Studies have indicated a slightly greater yield and slightly decreased follicular transection rate with microscopes over other methods of magnification. There have been no studies which indicate if this results in a difference in the outcome for the patient though. Magnification is the key to dissection. Loupe magnification is available which is as powerful as some microscopes. Ensuring that some type of magnification is used is essential to ensuring the best results.

Consultation

The consultation is the time for the patient to become familiar with the physician's practice, develop a rapport with the physician, and receive a diagnosis and treatment plan. It is not the time for high pressure sales pitches. Any treatment relies on a specific diagnosis and for patients contemplating hair transplants informed consent is vital before undertaking a procedure. Any consultation must include a visit with a physician. While consultants can be excellent resources to introduce patients to a physician's practice and inform patients about routines before and after surgery, only a physician can ensure that a patient has an accurate diagnosis of the cause of the patient's hair loss and an accurate treatment plan.

Patients should be careful of physicians who simply do whatever the patient asks. Often patient expectations for hair restoration surgery are not what will produce the best result. Part of the consultation should be about education of the hair loss process and methods for ensuring that hair restoration surgery will look natural for decades and not just months.

Fellowships

There are no fellowships certified by the American Board of Medical Specialties or any of its member boards. Physicians may advertise that they did a fellowship in hair restoration but this often reflects a time under the tutelage of someone who performs hair restoration. Since there is no accrediting organization there is no method to determine if standards are maintained or if the fellowship is teaching the current technology.

Facility and Equipment

Most hair restoration procedures are performed in a physician's office. This is very safely done but a couple of pitfalls must be pointed out. There are no national organizations which certify a physician's office as safe and in compliance with industry standard safety principles. Although hair restoration surgery has very few serious risks, anytime anything is injected into the body and surgical procedures are undertaken, there is the risk of allergic reactions. Instruments are often reused and must be sterilized between uses. To ensure that you are in a safe environment, ensure that your physician and his office have at least basic safeguards. These basic safeguards include:

- Autoclave with regular spore testing for sterility
- Protocols for cleaning equipment between patients
- If multiple procedures are performed at the same time, protocols for ensuring that donor hair is not mixed between patients
- Basic life support and/or advanced life support current certification for the physician and his staff
- Oxygen
- Defibrillator
- Advanced life support medications

Having an autoclave is important, but ensuring that it is functioning correctly with regular spore testing is essential. The testing is usually carried out by outside laboratories and your physician should be able to produce a log or other evidence that routine testing is being performed.

The physician and his staff should be trained in basic life support protocols through the American Heart Association and have the basic equipment necessary to deal with medical emergencies until paramedics can arrive. Simply knowing what to do without the proper tools is useless.

Second Opinion

As you will read in the advertising pitfalls section, there are very few, if any, procedures in the world which are performed by only one surgeon. It is wise to obtain a second opinion, especially about hair restoration procedures where diagnosis and design of the treatment plan are probably more important than the technical skill of the surgeon. Be careful though and make sure if you are shopping price that you are comparing apples to apples (more discussion in the Advertising Pitfalls section).

Suggested Questions to Ask Your Physician

What is your educational background?

This should include not only residency programs but also specialized training in hair restoration surgery.

Are you board certified?

As discussed, there is no board which certifies hair restoration surgeons. Importance should be placed on finding a physician certified in surgery with education in cosmetic and reconstructive facial surgery.

Where do you have hospital privileges?

As discussed above, hospital privileges are important should an untoward reaction occur.

What parts of the procedure do you perform and what do you delegate to your technicians?

Hair technicians are vital in hair restoration surgery - but physicians are absolutely key. After all, you are allowing the procedure to be performed by the physician, not the technicians. Setting up the ground rules in advance can save disaster later.

What life support equipment and training do you have?

Ensuring that your physician has both the training and equipment to deal with emergencies should they occur can be life saving.

What method of anesthesia do you use?

Be sure to address the method of anesthesia with your surgeon. If you think that local anesthesia will not be enough for you, ask your surgeon if she is comfortable with other types of anesthesia. The type of anesthesia will also dictate if you need a driver, what you can eat before the surgery, and if you need help after surgery.

Part XVII

Advertising Pitfalls

Because of the large amount of money to be made with hair loss treatments, competition is fierce. This necessitates large budgets for advertising. Unfortunately, all advertising must be looked at under a microscope. After all, the advertising is designed to wow a person into coming into the office to be sold something. Physicians are held to a higher standard in advertising than the general public. Unlike corporations which have civil laws to abide by, physicians have the same laws plus additional laws created by each state's medical boards. Drugs companies are also held to a high advertising standard as their advertising is also policed by the US Food and Drug Administration. Unfortunately not all cosmetic advertising is performed by physicians or drug companies. While most advertising by physicians is very reputable, some can be misleading. Patients must take all of the advertising in stride. This section aims to help identify some of the pitfalls of common advertising techniques so that appropriate scrutiny can be made of the advertising.

Before and After Photographs

Before and after photographs can be an excellent guide to a physician's results but must be taken with several words of warning.

- The photographs should be taken with the same background, the same lighting, and with the same camera and lens. In the age of digital photography, the photographs should also be taken with the same resolution settings. Photographs which are taken with different backgrounds and different lighting can produce various shadows which can slightly alter results.

- Make sure that the photographs are taken at the same angle, with the same head position, and the same hairstyle. Simply changing a hairstyle can give the perception of increased hair density and improvement even without actual improvement.

- Don't dismiss a surgeon simply because they do not have before and after photographs, especially when it comes to facial surgery. Photographs of patients must be used with their express written consent. Patients undergoing cosmetic surgery, even hair restoration, especially of the face, are often reluctant to allow their identifiable photographs to be used for everyone to see.

- Remember – photographs cannot be verified. With today's technology it is possible to alter images to take out blemishes imperceptibly.

- Most before and after photographs only show a physician's best results. Consider looking at a *consecutive* series of before and after photographs. While it is difficult to get a consecutive series of patients who are willing to use their photographs, 5-10 sets of photographs is optimal to really illustrate a physician's results. In this way, you won't just see the best that a physician has to offer but you will see the most likely results and possibly some less than optimal results.

- Remember that everyone is different. Before and after photographs illustrate the results obtained for a specific patient. This means a specific person's problem, their specific genetic makeup, their specific skin complexion, their specific medical problems, their specific postoperative course, and their specific procedures. Even though a physician performs the exact same procedure with the exact same technical skill, they may not get the exact same results.

- Determine if the photographs are those taken of the physician's patients or if the photographs are provided by a national company. Though the results may be great, they may not represent the ability of the specific physician to perform the procedure.

Testimonials

Testimonials can be very compelling statements. To hear another patient extol the virtues of a physician is very heart warming. Unfortunately the biggest drawback to a testimonial is that it cannot be verified. The testimonial can be completely fabricated or can be altered from the original context. There is no way to tell. Several states have limitations on the types of testimonials which can be made and advertised. Assuming the veracity of the testimonial, it will represent one person's experience. Given a physician sees several hundred people a year, this may not represent an accurate cross section of the practice. This applies to both positive and negative testimonials.

Speaking directly with a patient who has had a hair transplant with the surgeon you are considering can be helpful. This can help to ensure the truth behind any testimonial. Unfortunately, this too can be misleading. Remember that patients who agree to speak with other patients are generally chosen by the physician because they had a good experience, were pleased with their results, and are going to speak well of the physician. No physician would give out the names of patients who were unhappy with their service. Additionally, you may speak to one or two patients. This is not an adequate cross section of the entire practice.

Don't discount a physician who cannot provide referral patients. Hair transplants are cosmetic procedures most often performed on men who are not interested in making it known that they have had cosmetic surgery. It can be quite difficult to find patients who are willing to talk about their experience with others.

The "X" Procedure

There are many procedures in medicine which have been repackaged and marketed under a different name. Beware of procedures which are marketed as proprietary and being performed by a limited number of surgeons. If a procedure has stood the test of time and is a good procedure, it will be written about in the medical literature. As such, any physician will have access to how the procedure is performed and the procedure could be performed by more than a few surgeons. When you hear about a new procedure, visit http://www.pubmed.org and search for the procedure. At times the procedure will be listed under another generic name but pubmed should be able to find the procedure. Generally abstracts are available for free and you can purchase access to the entire scientific article. Procedures which produce good results will have peer reviewed scientific studies which bear out the results.

Free Consultations

Free consultations can be an excellent way to become acquainted with a physician's practice but they can also be a good way to get a high powered sales pitch. In some practices the physician will perform the consultation directly. In these cases, it can be a very informative session and often worth much more than it costs.

In other situations, patients may be evaluated solely by a 'consultant.' These consultants are often untrained personnel whose job it is to turn prospects into patients. In some situations these consultants are paid commissions based on the number of patients who undergo procedures. At times, patients may not be able to even see the physician until a deposit is paid and they agree to undergo surgery. In these situations, patients may not be the best candidates for the procedures for which they sign up.

In other contexts, there is a mix of a visit with a consultant and the physician. Consultants can be very helpful in educating patients about procedures and the practice flow of a physician's office. In the end, there is no substitute for a trained and experienced physician who can evaluate a patient and determine if they are an appropriate candidate for the procedure they are wishing to undergo.

Cosmetic surgery is costly. If you are serious about spending these large sums of money, paying $100-$200 for an extended visit with a physician should not be a primary concern.

Voted Best

Most 'Voted Best' physicians are very reputable. Unfortunately, the criteria for being 'voted best' is not always clear and can at times be misleading. When considering a 'voted best' physician, determine the criteria for voting and who bestowed the ranking. Was the voting done by a verified ballot or was it anonymous? Anonymous voting can lead to ballot stuffing by certain individuals. Was there a verification of the physician's credentials as part of the balloting? Some physicians may be voted 'best' but not have the training to perform the procedures they are being voted for. Were ballots mailed out or did it rely on people sending in votes? If ballots were mailed out, a more representative sample of results is available. If voting relied on people sending in votes, voting campaigns can be undertaken to sway the balloting. Does publication of names rely on purchasing of advertising? Some 'voted best' publications rely on the person being voted to buy advertising. For a reliable list, advertising should not be required.

Just because a physician is not in a 'best of' list does not mean they are not a good physician. Many excellent physicians are never 'voted best'.

The Latest Technology

Just because something is the latest, doesn't mean it is the greatest. Many technologies that have promising starts end up being removed from the market or improved after extended follow up because of unexpected long term results. In addition, companies which are new to a market may not last the test of time. One example of this is Artefill®. Artefill® was approved as a permanent facial filler in October of 2006. Unfortunately in November 2008, the manufacturer of Artefill®, Artes Medical filed for Chapter 7 bankruptcy.

This does not mean that the latest technology is a bad thing. For some things, the latest technology brings a fresh alternative with excellent results. At some point, all procedures were new. Waiting a year or two to determine long term results is never a bad idea before undertaking a new procedure.

Sometimes the old way is the best way. Consider a physician who performs both classic procedures and has access and knowledge of the latest technology. Patients will often get the best results from physicians who are able to take the best of the old and combine it with the latest techniques.

Awards

Physicians will often report on awards they have received from companies, report that they are on teaching faculty for certain companies, or they have received special training with certain certifications. While these can be well deserved and reflect outstanding performance, some are given for less ideal reasons. Some awards with fancy names are given by companies simply for purchasing a certain amount of product or attending a company sponsored training seminar. These awards do not reflect the ability of the physician to perform a procedure but rather reflect their willingness to invest in a certain product or procedure. If you see one of these rewards, be sure to ask the physician what it takes to receive the reward. Just because a physician buys X amount of product, doesn't mean that they can use that same product well and get the results that you expect.

Teaching faculty for companies are selected by the companies not necessarily based on the most competent physician available. These physicians are often compensated by the company for their time and receive travel compensation for special training sessions. While teaching faculty can be very good at what they do, it is not necessarily their competence which has gotten them to their position. At times, these faculty have come to the attention of the company for the amount of product which they are purchasing and not necessarily their ability to use the product correctly.

Some physicians will advertise that they have special training and special 'certifications.' While some of these certifications are issued by competent authorities, some are issued as a result of paying a fee or taking an online or weekend course. They do not necessarily reflect the competence of the physician or that the physician's ability to perform a procedure well has been tested. Finding a physician who is board certified and has received extensive training in a certain procedure is necessary to ensure that you get the best results possible. For a full discussion of board certification, please read the section on Choosing Your Physician.

Over 1,000 Performed

Determining how many of a procedure a physician has performed is always a good idea. For some things, more is better. For others, more is not necessarily better. Just because a physician has performed 10,000 procedures in a year, doesn't mean that he is the best at it or that he will get the results that you desire. 10,000 bad results are still 10,000 results.

Be careful too of the large corporations which extoll having performed thousands of procedures. Facial rejuvenation procedures aren't like Big Macs®, one isn't like the next. Each must be individualized and the results are partly based on the skill of the surgeon performing the procedure. Though there may have been thousands performed by the corporation, each physician may not have performed thousands.

Special Pricing

While special pricing can provide excellent value for patients, be ware of specials which exist only for a day or packages which require you to pay for an entire series of treatments in advance to get the best price. When considering hair restoration procedures, the best price may not create the best result. In some situations, the best price may turn into a much more costly experience if revision procedures are necessary because the original procedure was performed by a provider who was less than qualified.

Be sure to read the fine print. Sometimes package pricing or high pressure sales can require putting down a large sum of money which is nonrefundable even if you decide to only perform one or two procedures or none at all. Be especially careful if you have to finance the procedures. Be sure to read all of the fine print in the financing documents before deciding to proceed. Even if you can get back the money for your deposit, you may still owe interest and penalties to the financing company.

Understanding Pricing

In an ideal world, medical treatment should not be about price. Unfortunately, economic reality is that patients often shop for the best deal when considering hair restoration surgery. To adequately 'shop', patients must understand the pricing that physicians are offering. The first step in the education process is to make sure everyone is talking the same language. Two terms often talked about with hair transplants are grafts and hairs. Grafts refer to a collection of follicular units. This can mean that anywhere from 1-6 hairs may be transplanted in one graft. On the other hand, hair refers to individual hairs. Some physicians may only transplant individual hairs so that grafts and hairs are interchangeable. Patients should ask their physicians how many hairs will be transplanted as well as how many grafts. If they are the same number, this indicates that individual hair grafts will be placed. While this is adequate for the hairline, it will take many more grafts to provide density than if multi unit grafts are used.

Pricing is generally divided into three categories:

- Per session
- Per graft
- Per hair

Some physicians may provide a combination of pricing structures. For instance, the physician may charge X dollars for the first session which provides up to Y grafts and each additional graft will cost Z dollars.

Though the exact cost of a transplant will often depend on exactly how many hairs are transplanted, physicians should be able to provide you with an estimate of the cost. Ask for the estimate based on total number of hairs AND total number of grafts. This way you should be able to more easily compare prices from different physicians.

Another word of caution, determine what your physician's cost is for additional hair transplant sessions. For some patients, multiple sessions will be required to obtain optimal results. Be sure to determine what your physician's policy is for these additional sessions. Again, getting a total price for your plan is best. This includes total number of hairs, total number of grafts, and total number of sessions. This will help to balance the field when comparing prices.

Hair Transplant Affiliations

Many physicians will advertise that they are a member of various hair societies. As mentioned, there is no ABMS board which certifies hair transplant surgeons. Physicians can be members of various organizations which are dedicated to education about hair restoration surgery. While membership does indicate a physicians interest in the procedure and dedication to furthering their knowledge, do not confuse membership with any kind of credentialing process. Membership often requires only paying an annual fee and filling out an application. There are several hair restoration organizations which provide education not only for physicians but also for patients. These include:

- International Society of Hair Restoration Surgery
- American Society of Hair Restorations Surgeons
- World Hair Society
- The American Hair Loss Council
- The American Hair Loss Association
- The International Alliance of Hair Restoration Surgeons

Just because a physician is a member of these organizations does not signify any special ability, simply an interest in the procedure.

FDA Approved

FDA approval and FDA clearance are designations provided by the United States Food and Drug administration to show that a product has been through clinical studies and proven safe and effective compared to some benchmark. While approval and clearance are two completely different processes, suffice it to say that clinical evidence needs to be presented to obtain the ability to advertise FDA clearance or approval. FDA clearance and approval are specific to devices and medications. Just because one specific device has FDA clearance, doesn't mean that all similar devices have FDA clearance.

While the FDA does police companies that say that they are FDA cleared or approved and have limitations on advertising, it is more of a retroactive policing, relying on reports of abuse. To determine if a device or medication is FDA cleared or approved, visit http://www.fda.gov. There are sections for devices and sections for medications which indicate exactly what the indications for each of the cleared or approved devices is.

Be careful, some devices make the claim that they are FDA approved when they are not. In fact, similar devices may be FDA approved but the particular device is not. In addition, be ware of what companies claim as their approval. FDA approval or clearance is for a very specific indication, such as 'hair loss for male patients between 18 and 65.' More general claims should be a red flag requiring verification with the US FDA.

Additional Web References

http://www.ishrs.org
http://www.ahlc.org
http://www.iahrs.org

Web sites for various hair transplant organizations

http://www.fda.gov

The official site of the United States Food and Drug Administration which can be used to verify FDA clearance or approval for devices and medications.

Part XVIII

F.A.Q.

Frequently Asked Questions

These frequently asked questions about hair restoration surgery are taken from my web site. While the text of the book has significantly more detail, this section will provide quick answers for common questions about current hair restoration surgery technology.

Will my final result look like plugs in my scalp?

No. Older techniques produced results which look like plugs in the scalp. New techniques of micrografting and minigrafting result in a natural looking hairline.

Will I need to be asleep for the procedure?

No. The procedures are performed on an outpatient basis with only local anesthesia. Occasionally a patient prefers mild sedation and we can accommodate such requests.

Is the procedure painful?

There is some discomfort associated with the procedure. This usually subsides by the second day after surgery. You will be given a prescription pain medicine. Most patients just take this on the day of surgery. Tylenol usually takes care of any discomfort after the first day.

Where will the procedure be performed?

The procedures are performed in our office. We have a procedure room and specialized equipment just for our hair restoration patients. Bring a DVD of a movie you would like to watch, pick from our limited selection, or just watch a little cable television. We ask that you not wear earphones as thy can be soiled during the procedure.

How long will surgery take?

Depending on the number of grafts and the degree of baldness, surgery may take anywhere from 4-14 hours. You will have breaks during that time however.

How long do I have to take it easy?

We ask that you avoid strenuous activity for one week after the procedure. This will prevent bleeding and aid the healing process.

When will I start to see results?

New hair growth will not start for 4 to 6 months. Prior to this, stubble will fall out and the grafts will look bare. This is completely normal. Most of all, be patient during the healing process. The results will be well worth the wait.

When can I return to work?

Most people are able to return to work the day after the procedure. You will have some small red dots where the hairs are transplanted but these can be easily covered with a ball cap.

What is the ideal age for a hair transplant?

There is no ideal age for a hair transplant. The important thing to remember is what the expected balding pattern of the person is before they get a transplant. Balding will continue even after a transplant. If the surgeon is not careful he can create a hairline which will look unnatural as further hair loss occurs. This can then produce a very difficult problem if the donor site is already used.

Should I take medications after my transplant?

Yes. It would be a very good idea to start on Finasteride (Propecia®) or Minoxidil (Rogaine®) around the time of your transplant. It will not grow back hair that you have lost but it will slow the progression of hair loss.

Will the transplanted thin as my natural hair does?

No. The donor site is taken from an area which does not fall out. When transplanted, it retains this property and will not fall out even in its new location. It is important to note though that hair loss will progress. This can result in a thinning even in the transplanted area from a loss of the native hair in that area.

Will I be black and blue with bruising and swelling?

While every patient is different, bruising and swelling are usually minimal. You will notice that over the course of the first week after surgery, you will have swelling that will go from your scalp to your forehead and down to around your eyes. This usually subsides very quickly.

Will I have to wear bandages on my head?

No. You will have no bandages of any kind. In fact, we want you to leave the transplanted area open to the air as much as possible. We suggest that you do not wear a hairpiece for a month around the time of surgery but will work with you if this is a problem.

Will I have to have sutures removed?

You will have sutures at the donor site. If you live near the office we will schedule to see you in 10-14 days for suture removal. This is a simple process and is not painful. If you live far from the office we can either help you to arrange for them to be removed in 10-14 days or we can use dissolvable sutures which will fall out on their own in about 3-4 weeks.

When can I drive?

You can drive yourself home. As long as you do not require more than the normal amount of anesthesia you can drive yourself home. It is extremely unusual for people to want sedation for this procedure, but if you elect to have sedation, you will need a driver to and from the procedure.

Index

Symbols

A

B

C

D

E

F

G

H

I

J

L

M

N

O

P

R

S

T

U

V

W

Y

Z

www.ingramcontent.com/pod-product-compliance
Lightning Source LLC
LaVergne TN
LVHW091010080826
845145LV00003B/1215

* 9 7 8 0 5 7 8 0 1 4 9 2 0 *